Bridal Hair

Pat Dixon and Jacki Wadeson

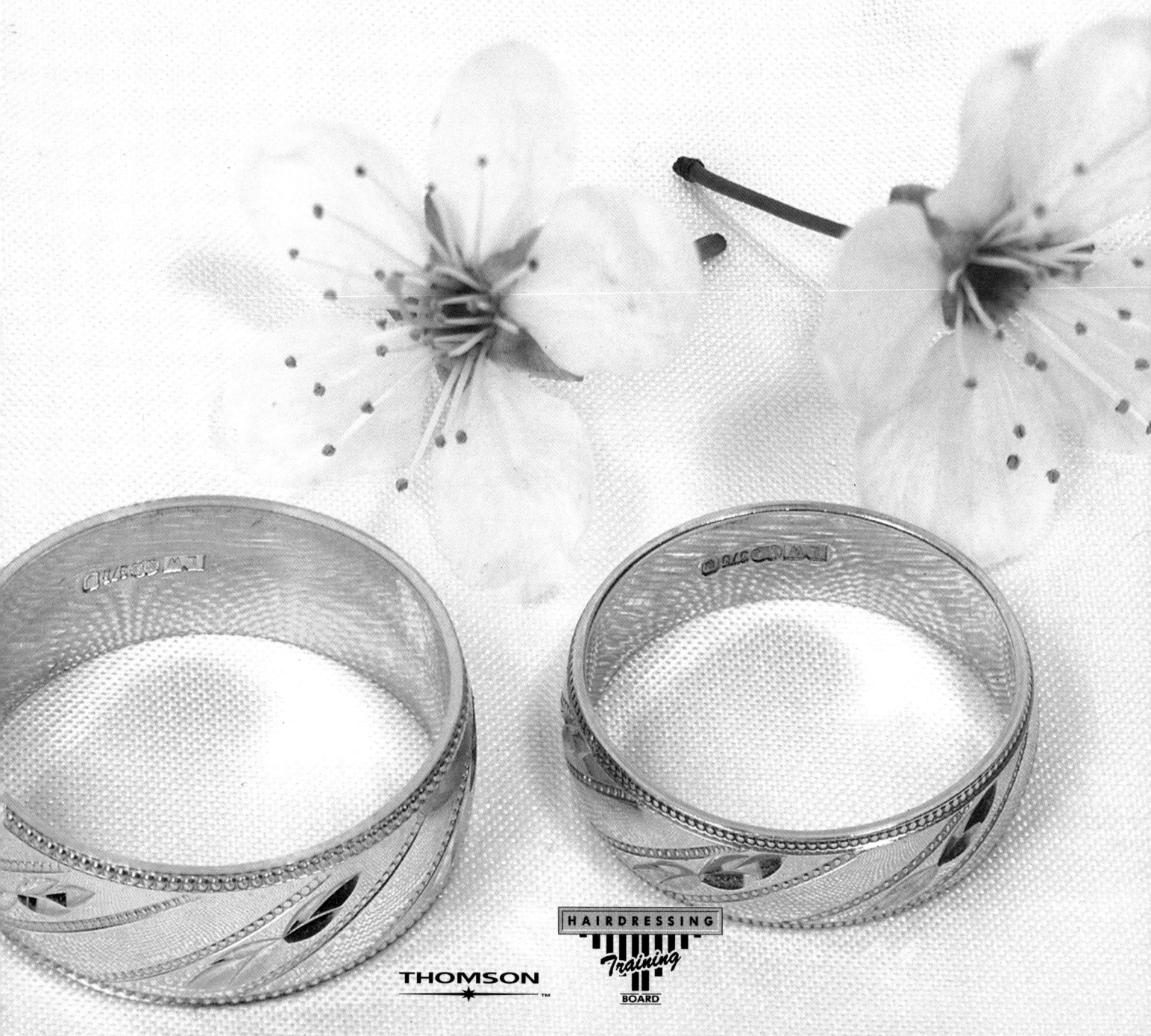

THOMSON

HAIRDRESSING Training BOARD

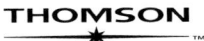

Bridal Hair

For more information, contact Thomson Learning, High Holborn House; 50-51 Bedford Row, London WC1R 4LR or visit us on the World Wide Web at:
http://www.thomsonlearning.co.uk

British Library Cataloguing-in-Publication Data
A catalogue record for this book is available from the British Library

ISBN 1-86152-893-0

First published in 2000 by MacMillan Press Ltd

This version printed 2002 by Thomson Learning
Reprint 2003 by Thomson Learning

Printed digitally in Croatia by Zrinski d.d.

Contents

Hairdressing Training Board / Thomson Series

Start Hairdressing! – The Official Guide to Level 1 Martin Green & Leo Palladino

Hairdressing: The Foundations – The Official Guide to Level 2 Leo Palladino

Professional Hairdressing – The Official Guide to Level 3 Martin Green, Lesley Kimber & Leo Palladino

Patrick Cameron: Dressing Long Hair Patrick Cameron & Jacki Wadeson

Patrick Cameron: Dressing Long Hair Book 2 Patrick Cameron

Mahogany: Steps to Cutting, Colouring and Finishing Hair Martin Gannon & Richard Thompson

Safety in the Salon Elaine Almond

Trevor Sorbie: Visions in Hair Trevor Sorbie, Kris Sorbie & Jacki Wadeson

The Art of Hair Colouring David Adams & Jacki Wadeson

African-Caribbean Hairdressing Sandra Gittens

Men's Hairdressing Maurice Lister

Bridal Hair Pat Dixon & Jacki Wadeson

The Total Look Ian Mistlin

The Beauty Salon and its Equipment John V. Simmons

Manicure, Pedicure and Advanced Nail Techniques Elaine Almond

The Complete Make-up Artist: Working in Film, Television and Theatre Penny Delamar

The World of Skin Care John Gray

Beauty Therapy – The Foundations – The Official Guide to Level 2 Lorraine Nordmann

Professional Beauty Therapy – The Official Guide to Level 3 Lorraine Nordmann, Lorraine Appleyard & Pamela Linforth

Foreword

Do you create magic?

Can you imagine the perfect style?

A wedding is what you make it. For most people it's a special occasion, an opportunity for celebration. But for a bride it has to be the most special day in her life. And she expects her hair to be part of the magic of her special day.

As a professional hairdresser, you can weave your magic and produce the perfect style. This book contains a range of imaginative and aspirational styles that will widen your repertoire. Your brides will appreciate it.

Alan Goldsbro
Chief Executive
Hairdressing Training Board

Acknowledgements

Hair: Pat Dixon, Classics Hair & Beauty, Kenilworth

Step-by-step make-up: Liz Hoskins and the beauty staff at Classics Hair & Beauty, Kenilworth

Bridal style gallery make-up: Vicki Cameron, Carol Maye and Amanda Lawley

Photography: Simon Donnelly

Still-life photography: Barry Cook

Classics Bridal Hire Collection, 1 High Street, Kenilworth, CV8 1LY.
Tel: + 44 (0) 1926 511246

Cocoa, 9 Clarence Parade, Cheltenham, Gloucestershire, GL50 3NY.
Tel: + 44 (0) 1242 233588

Kesté by Myring Kesterton, Studio 209, The Custard Factory, Gibb Street,
Digbeth, Birmingham, B9 4AA. Tel: + 44 (0) 121 683 5108

Vicki Waring, 53 Wainbody Avenue, Coventry, CV3 6DA.
 Tel: + 44 (0) 1203 410098

The Flower Cellar, The Old Forge, Balsall Street, Balsall Common, Warwickshire,
CV7 7AP. Tel: + 44 (0) 1676 534117

Pauline Worthington at Cobwebs and Creations Jewellery Workshop.
Tel: + 44 (0) 1676 542284

Karen Singleton, 85 Coronation Road, Southville, Bristol, BS3 1AT.
Tel: + 44 (0) 117 9637474

Virgin Bride, The Grand Buildings, Northumberland Avenue, London WC2N 5EJ.
Tel: + 44 (0) 171 766 9112

Heapys Morning Suit Hire, Westgate House, Warwick, CV34 4DH.
Tel: + 44 (0) 1926 400647

H. Samuel, branches nationwide, call Freephone 0800 3894683

With special thanks to: Cara Wagstaff, Myring Kesterton, Vicki Waring, Carol Price, Pauline Worthington, Karen Singleton, Kim Baker, Caroline Neville Associates, Jane Bloxham, and all our beautiful models.

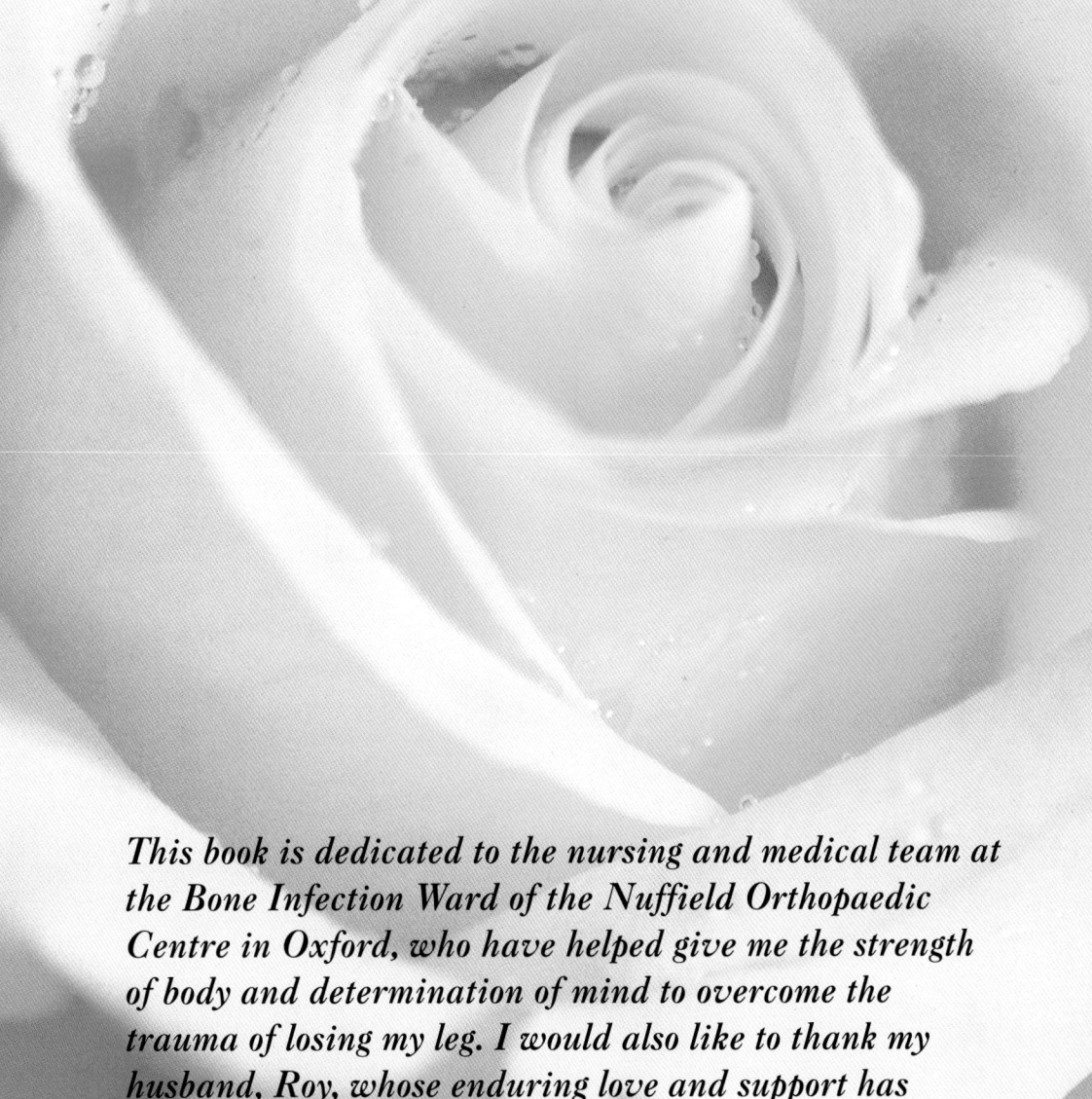

This book is dedicated to the nursing and medical team at the Bone Infection Ward of the Nuffield Orthopaedic Centre in Oxford, who have helped give me the strength of body and determination of mind to overcome the trauma of losing my leg. I would also like to thank my husband, Roy, whose enduring love and support has enabled me to continue my career in hairdressing.

Pat Dixon

Introduction

On the most important day of a bride's life, the only person who can create the hairstyle of her dreams is her hairdresser. This beautiful book explains how to offer a comprehensive bridal hair and beauty service: from helping your bride to choose her dress, head-dress and flowers to co-ordinating these with a style that suits her hair type and texture. Whatever her hair length, you and your bride will find inspiration in our bridal style gallery. Techniques, from the basic to the more complicated, are all illustrated in our easy-to-follow step-by-steps that fulfil many of the NVQ Levels 2 and 3 criteria. There is also a selection of romantic styles for seasonal and themed weddings, plus hints and tips on working with flowers, veils and hats. Everything you need to know to ensure that your bridal clients look magical on their wedding day.

Jacki Wadeson

Consultation

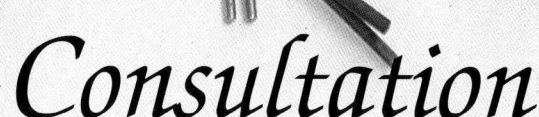

Ideally your bride should visit the salon three months before the wedding for a consultation of at least 30 minutes. It is a good idea if her mother or a friend accompanies her, and essential that she brings along details of the dress she has chosen or is planning to buy. You need to know whether the dress is simple or fussy, slim or full and, most importantly, what type of neckline it has. Hair tone and depth should also be taken into consideration when finalising the fabric and head-dress colour: white is good with ash-blonde, medium brown or black hair; colours from ivory to oyster go well with strawberry blonde, auburn or chestnut hair; gold looks good with warm hair tones such as golden brown, chestnut and red; silver suits dark blondes, blue-black, ash-brown or ash-blonde hair and pastels look best on fair hair.

Ask about the timing and type of wedding: Is it going to have a traditional, modern, classical or medieval theme? Is it going to be in a church or will it be a civil ceremony? Does the bride have definite ideas about whether she wants to wear a tiara, veil, flowers, diamanté clips, slides, pearls or butterflies in her hair?

Assess the bride's face and body shape so you can make sure the finished hairstyle balances perfectly. Check how tall the bridegroom is – you don't want to suggest a head-dress that leaves the bride towering over him. Have to hand a bridal style book containing pictures that show different looks so you can get a general feel of the bride's preferences. Once you have decided on the best style, then check whether the bride's hair type and texture are suitable. A beautiful head of tonged curls may be her romantic dream but if you know the hair will drop, persuade her to opt for something different. If a head-dress or veil is being worn, check its weight – it may not stay in place if the hair is too fine.

Make sure the bride has thought about her outfit as a whole; shoes and jewellery are important elements. The overall look should also be in keeping with her general style. Another consideration is whether the bride is going to change for an evening party. If so, her hair will need to be designed so that it will look good with both outfits.

Once you have decided on the best and most appropriate style, then is the time to draw up a pre-wedding hair and beauty plan, which includes a schedule to get hair healthy and glossy in time for the wedding. Include recommendations for timings of colour, cutting and perms, for facial, body and nail treatments, and for artificial tanning. Draw up a list of home maintenance products so the bride can keep up the good work between salon visits. Book an appointment for a dress rehearsal and find out whether the bride will visit the salon on the day or whether she wants her hair done on site. Don't forget the rest of the wedding party – the bride's mother, the bridesmaids and the bridegroom will also need to book salon appointments at this time.

Hair accessories: Classics Bridal Hire Collection and Virgin Bride

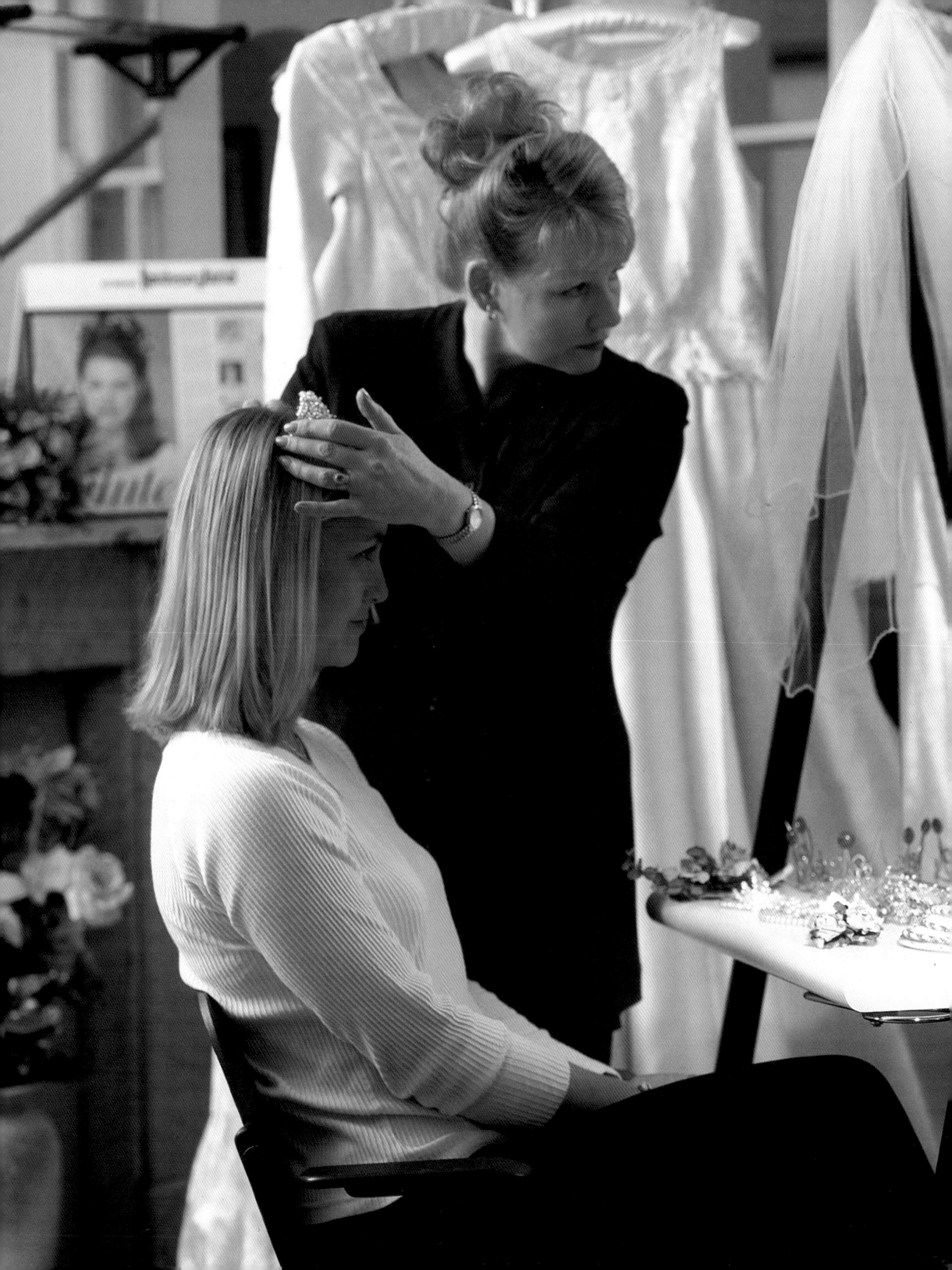

Head-dresses

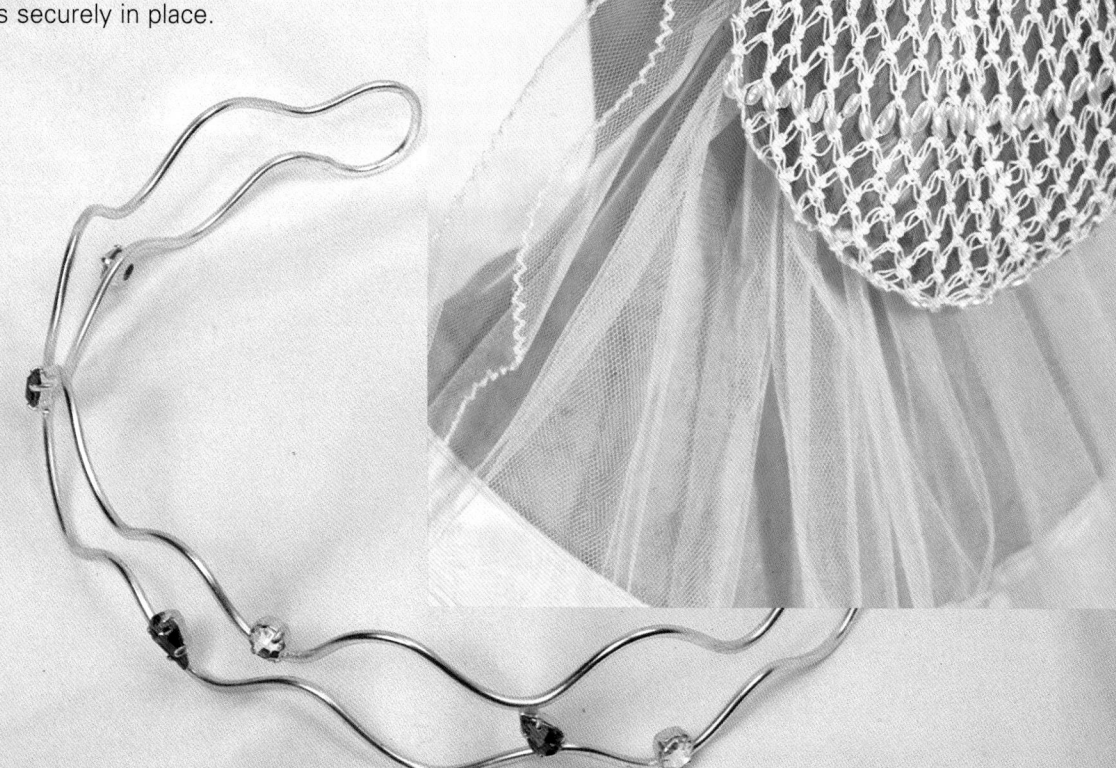

Head-dresses are a bride's crowning glory, and there are so many beautiful styles to choose from: close-fitting skullcaps, beaded combs, snoods, floral headbands, richly jewelled antique tiaras encrusted with crystals and diamanté or modern tiaras on more minimalist lines.

Many designers will custom-make head-dresses to suit the line and shape of the dress. If this is what your bride wants, then make sure she places her order in plenty of time.

Whichever head-dress is chosen, it is important to have a trial run. Don't rely on the combs or fixings that are already attached to the head-dress. Experiment with additional clips and pins to ensure it stays securely in place.

Snood and beaded comb: Classics Bridal Hire Collection
Headbands: Virgin Bride

Opposite Skullcap and dress: Cocoa

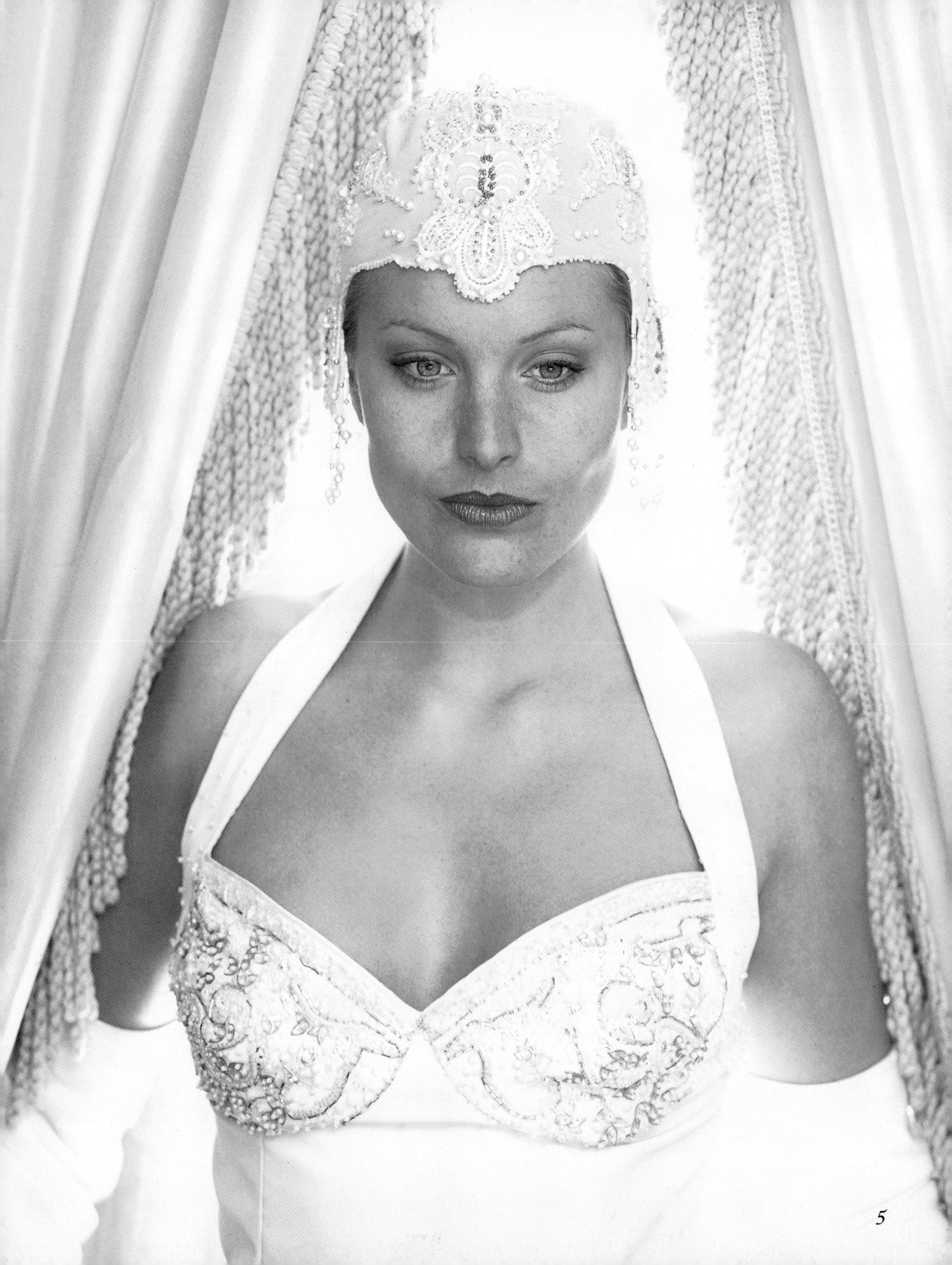

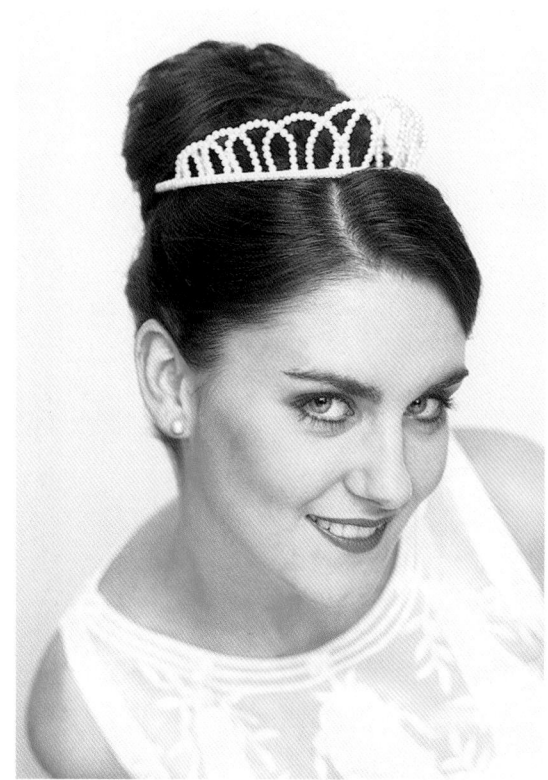

A simple upswept style can be changed by the choice of tiara – see how the purity of pearls gives a clean line, glamorous gems a richer look and glass stones set in gold a more regal air.

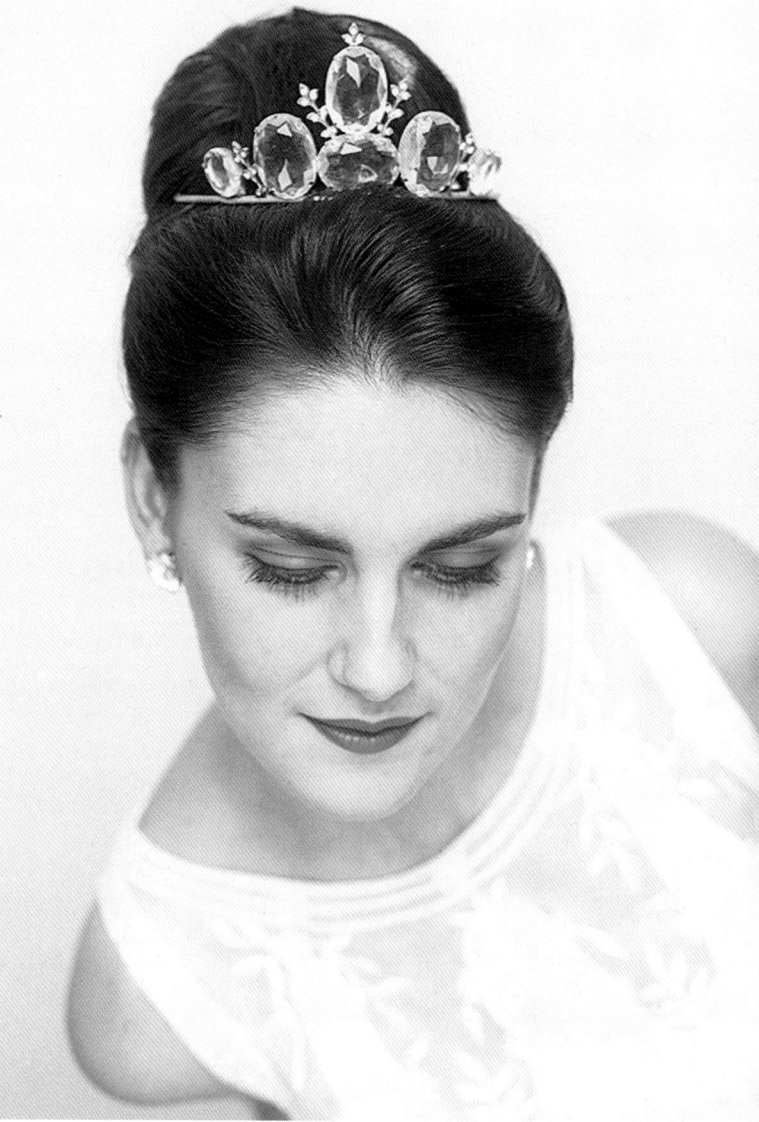

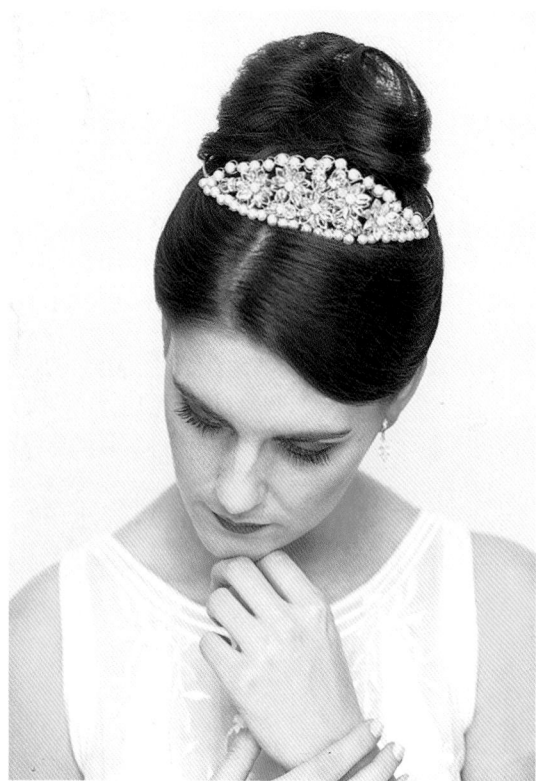

Dress and tiaras: Classics Bridal Hire Collection

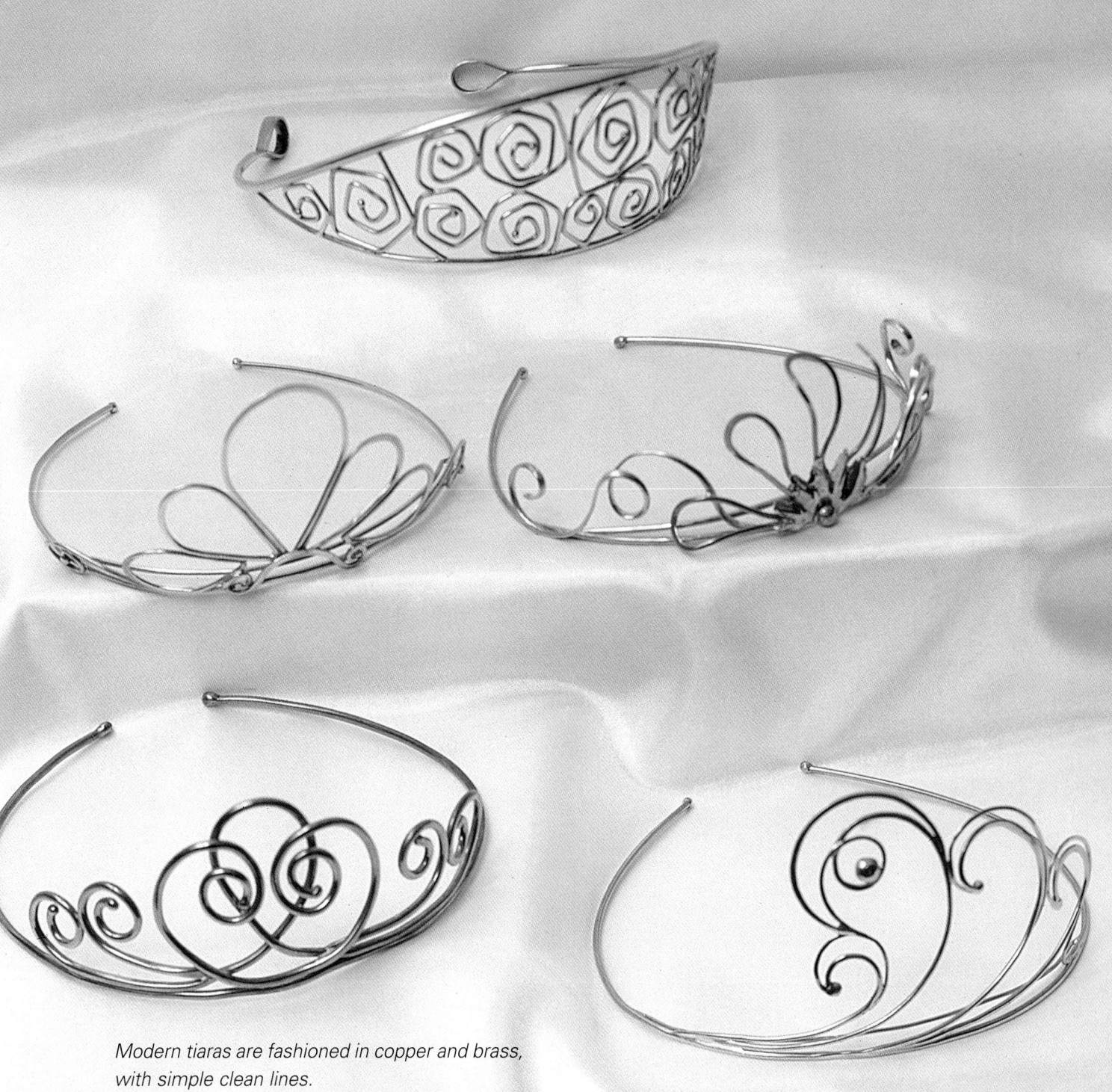

Modern tiaras are fashioned in copper and brass, with simple clean lines.

Modern tiaras: Cobwebs and Creations Jewellery Workshop

7

Antique tiaras are often very ornate with seed pearls, mother of pearl and an abundance of diamanté.

Antique tiaras and dress: Cocoa

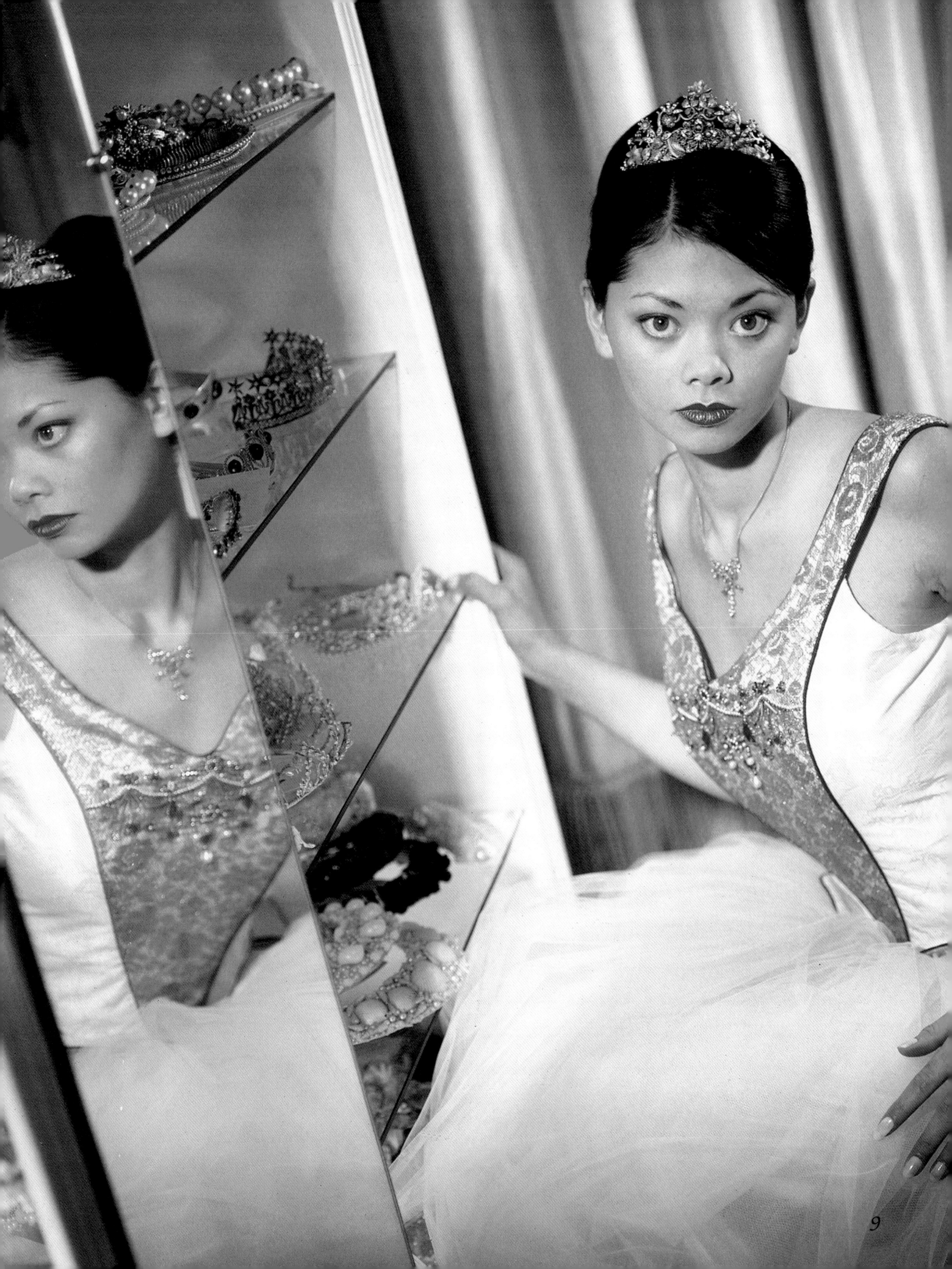

Flowers

Single flowers gripped into a hairstyle make an instant transformation. Keep blooms in a cool place before use and mist with water to freshen up before clipping into hair.

How to fix flowers in place

1 Thread stem of flower through looped end of a hairpin.

———— ✳ ————

2 Push hairpin into hair, then further secure flower stem with a hairgrip. Repeat with as many flowers as you wish to use.

———— ✳ ————

3 Shows side view.

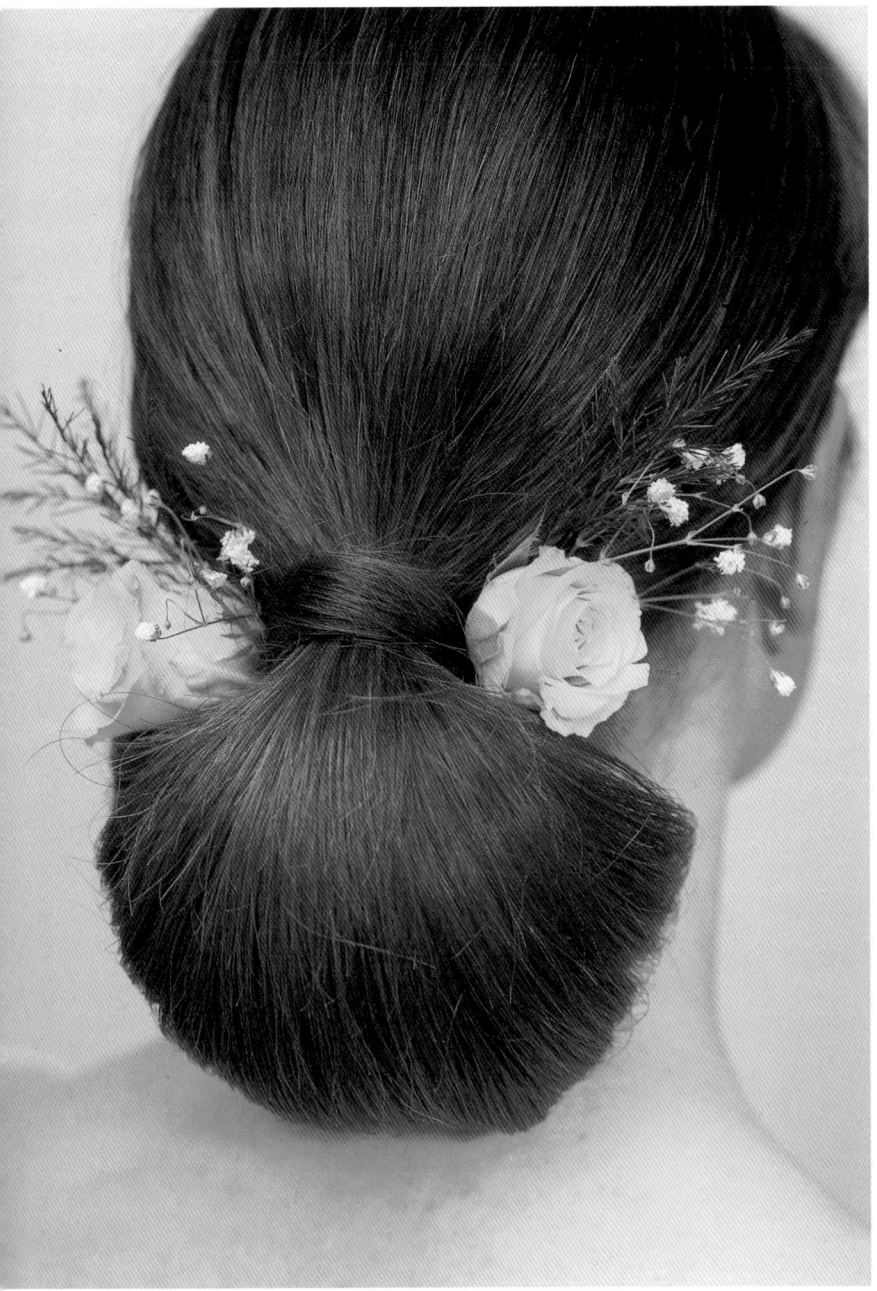

Roses and gypsophila gripped to either side of a low ponytail are simple yet effective.

Flowers: The Flower Cellar

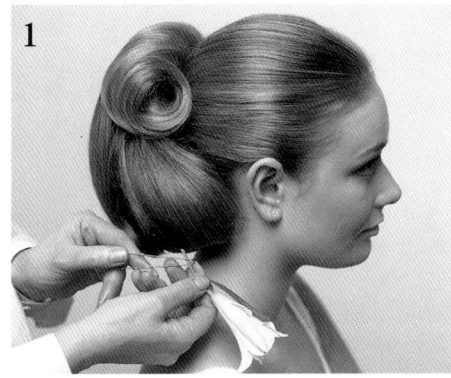

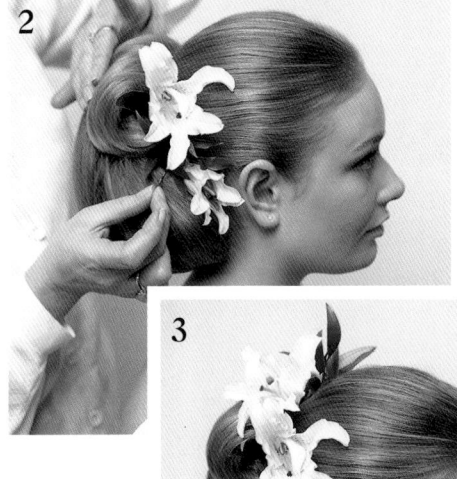

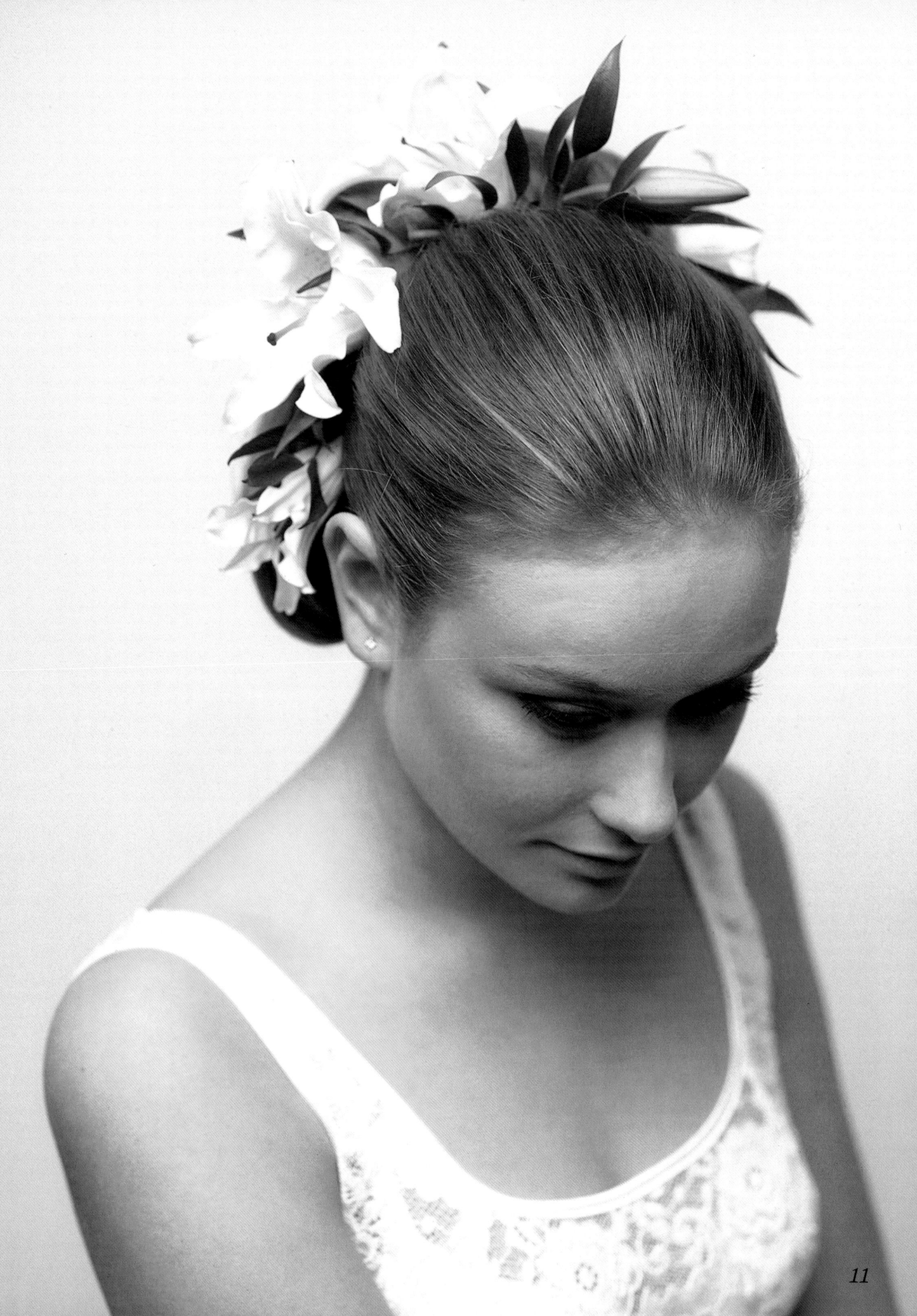

Veils

Veils add the finishing touch to the bride and give a fairytale aura to the simplest dress. The more layers the veil has, the fuller the look. Pure silk or antique veils have a softer feel and flow better than the stiffer man-made veiling or net. Embroidery, beading, ribboned edges and crystals draw attention to the veil. Opt for a simple veil with an ornate gown, or a more detailed one with a plain dress. Veils always work best when the hairstyle has some height, which gives lift and balance to the look. There are many different styles of veils. Five popular styles are listed opposite.

Bouffant – this just touches the shoulders and is quite fluffy and informal. Fun with shorter hair.

Cathedral – very long, this type of veil finishes six feet after the train. Looks beautiful with almost any hairstyle.

Church – full-length veil that ends about foot beyond the dress. Exquisite with more elaborate hairstyles.

Fingertip – ends where your fingertips touch your legs when you are standing. Perfect with soft curls or ringlets.

Mantilla – a lace-trimmed one-layer veil that frames the face and is attached with pins or a comb. Superb with smoother, dressier hairstyles.

How to secure a veil

1 Attach a hairgrip to each end of tiara and push into place.

——— ✳ ———

2 Insert comb which is attached to veil into hair and slide in until it feels firm.

——— ✳ ———

3 Take veil back over hair and fluff out.

——— ✳ ———

4 Shows veil and tiara in place.

TIP

To remove creases from a veil, hold taut and use the hot air from your hairdryer to smooth over the surface. Modern veils can be stiffened with spray starch but this is not suitable for antique ones as it may damage the fabric.

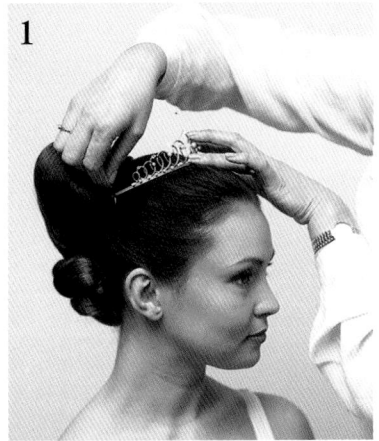

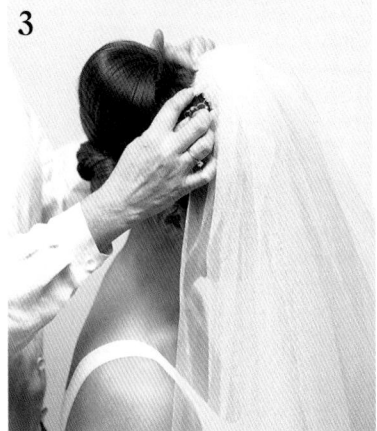

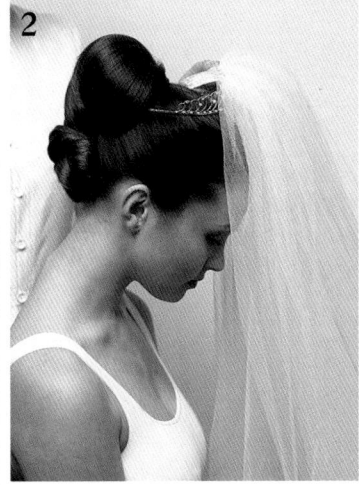

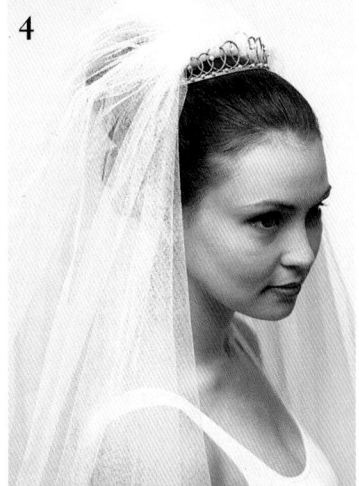

Opposite Dress, head-dress and hand-embroidered choker: Cocoa

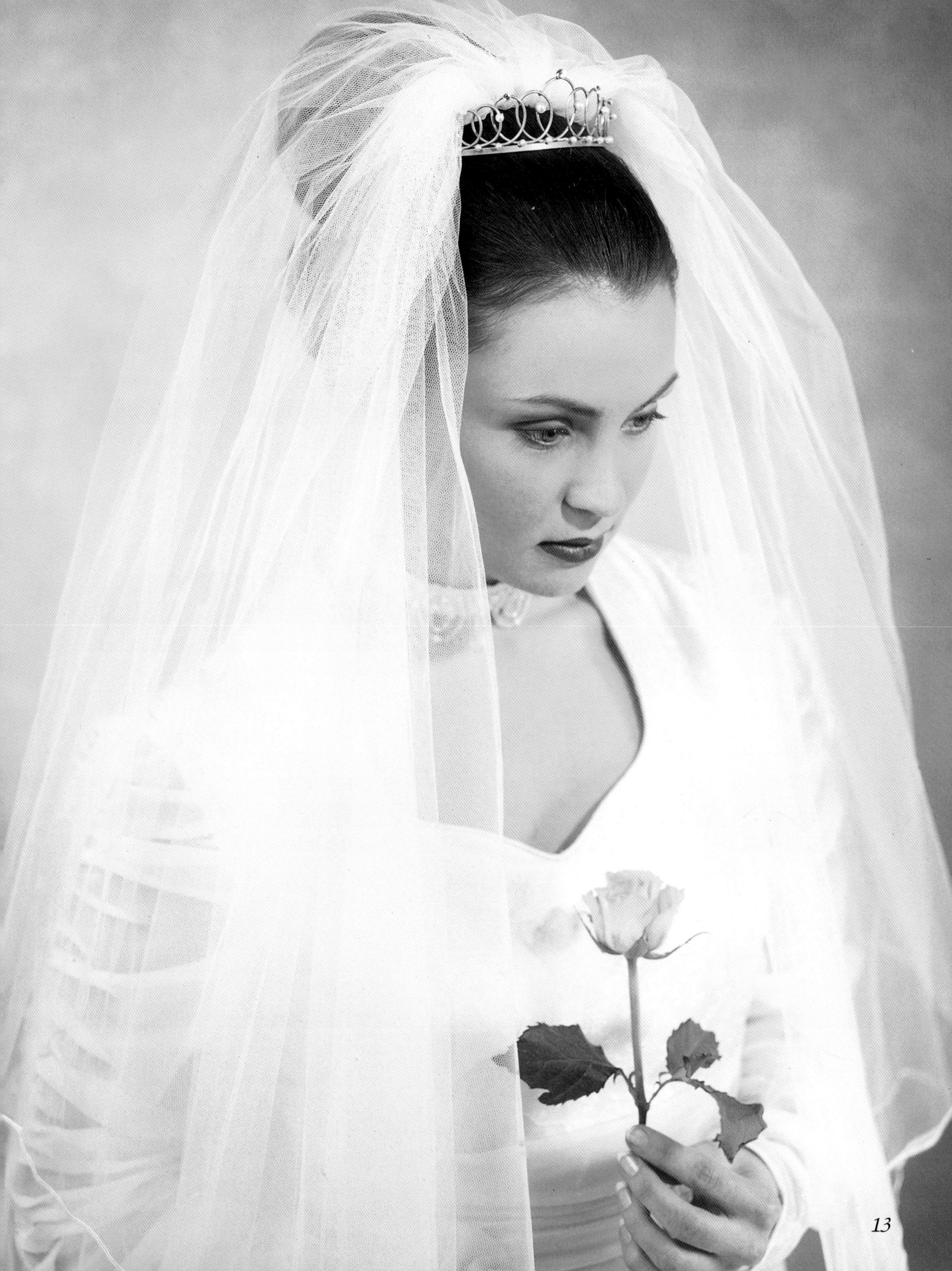

13

Hats

Hats are often the first choice for thirty-something brides who are having a civil wedding. Whether the design is plain, or swathed with organza, lace, or flowers, it needs a neat hairstyle that balances perfectly. Short hair can be styled behind the ears, while longer locks are best slicked back and formed into a neat, smooth bun at the nape of the neck.

How to dress hair to wear with a hat

1 Smooth hair back into a low ponytail. Divide hair into sections and wind onto heated rollers. Leave rollers in place until hair and rollers are completely cool.

——— ✳ ———

2 Remove rollers and take a small section of hair from underneath and wrap round base of ponytail. Pin in place.

——— ✳ ———

3 Shows back of hair completed before positioning hat.

> ### TIP
>
> When a hat is worn with longer hair, it is important that the ponytail is positioned low into the nape of the neck so that the hat sits perfectly.

1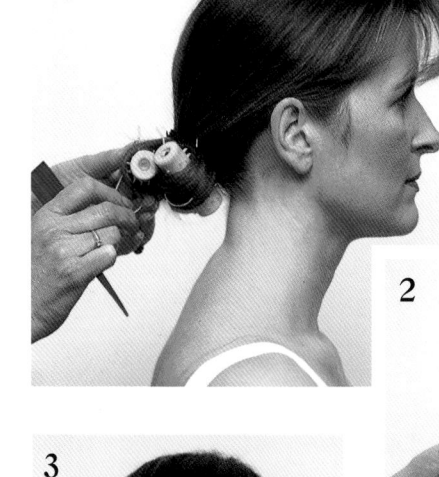

2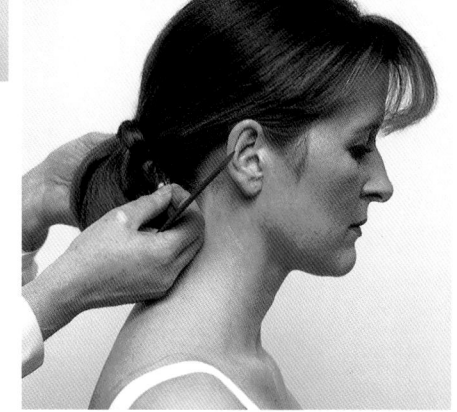

3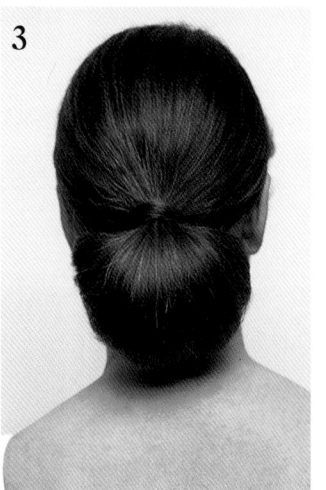

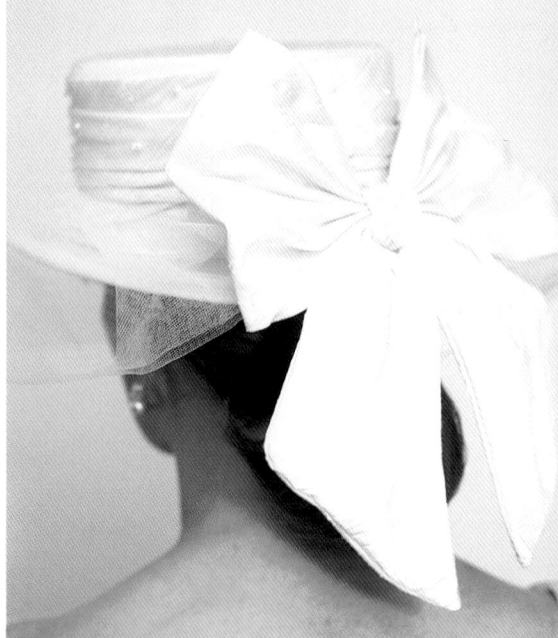

Opposite Dress and hat: Classics Bridal Hire Collection

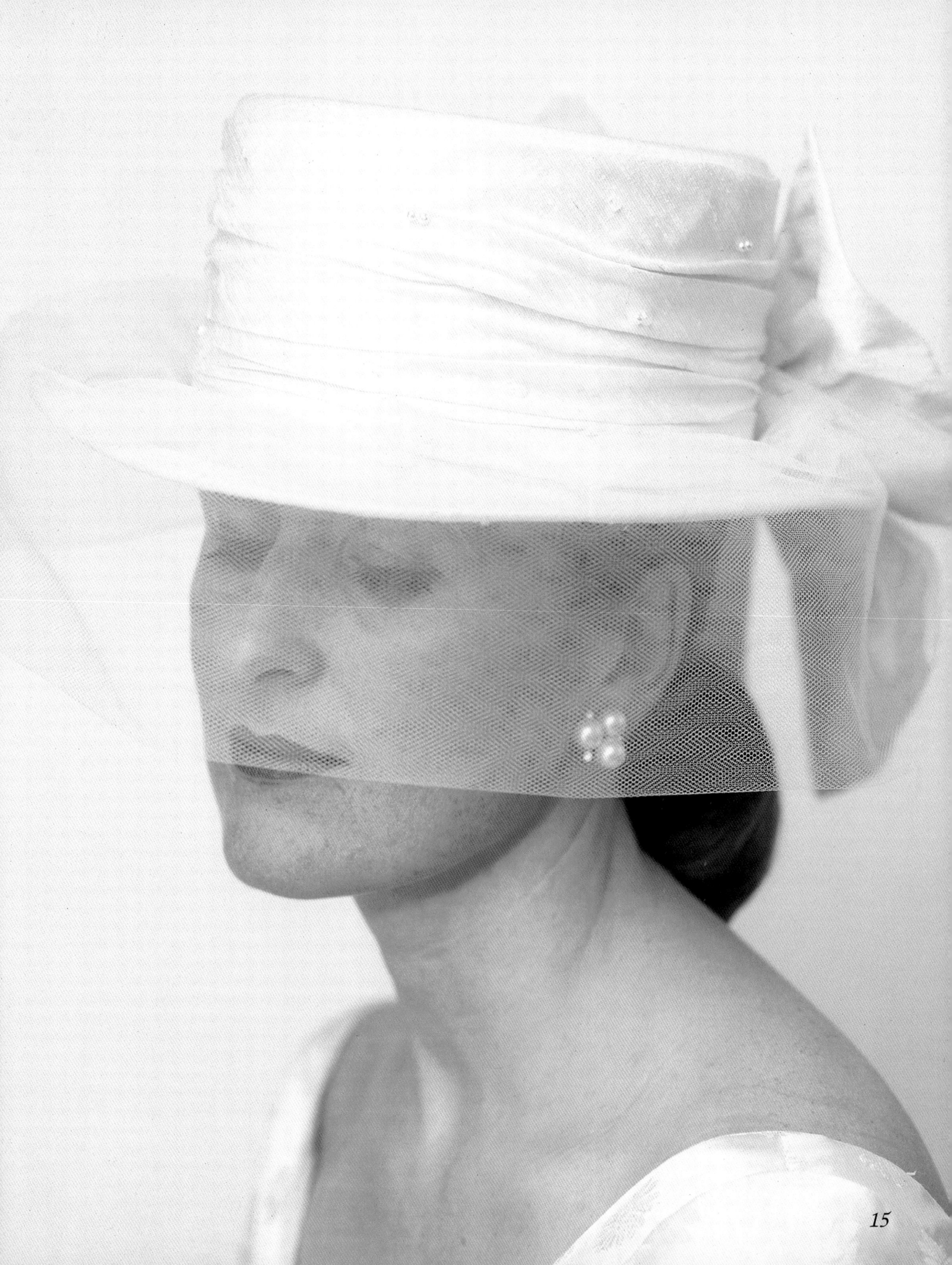

Bouquets

A wedding isn't complete without flowers, and these days brides have a wondrous array of blooms to choose from, most of which are available all year round. The key to getting perfect wedding flowers is to talk to the florist, who will be able to advise you as to what shape of bouquet will flatter the wedding gown. Flowers should complement, rather than overpower, the wedding outfit. Whether the bride chooses a trailing shower bouquet or a hand-held posy, it's important to keep things in proportion. As a general rule, the bigger the skirt the bigger the bouquet. Also, a tall bride can carry a larger bouquet than a petite bride.

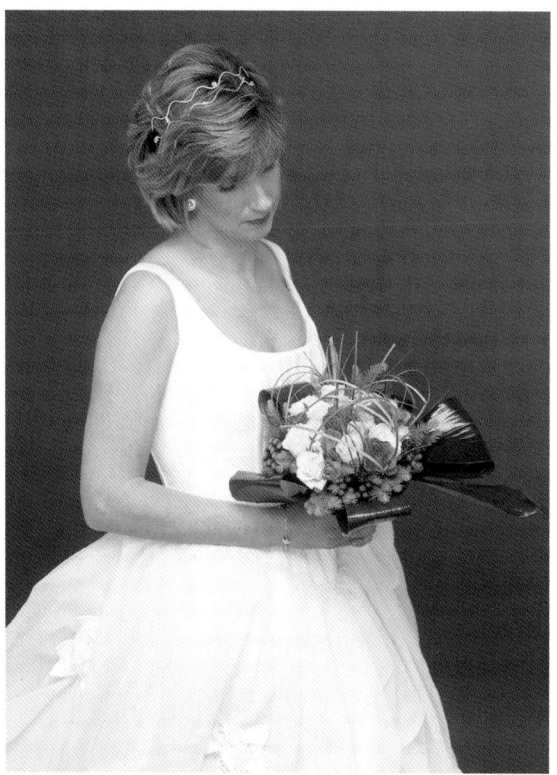

Dress and jewelled hairband: Virgin Bride
Flowers: The Flower Cellar

The meaning of flowers

Azalea – true to the end
Cedar leaf – I live for you
Celandine – joys to come
Chervil – sincerity
Forget-me-not – true love
Freesia – fragrant
Geranium – true friendship
Gorse – enduring affection
Heliotrope – devotion
Hyacinth – constancy
Ivy – fidelity
Mudwort – happiness
Pink – pure love
Red rose – love
Sweet pea – bright
Violet – faithfulness
White rose – purity

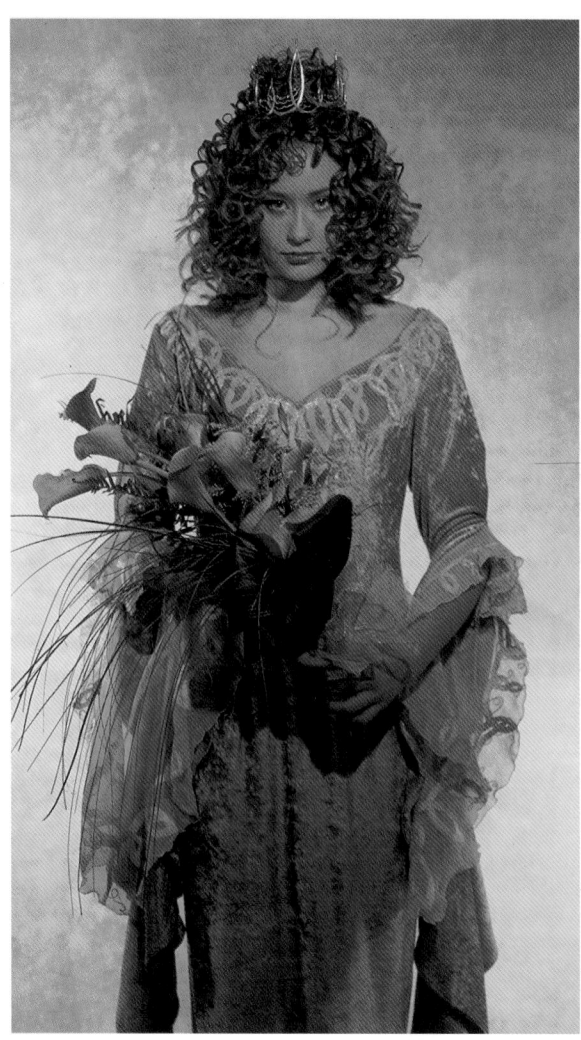

Dress and tiara: Kesté by Myring Kesterton

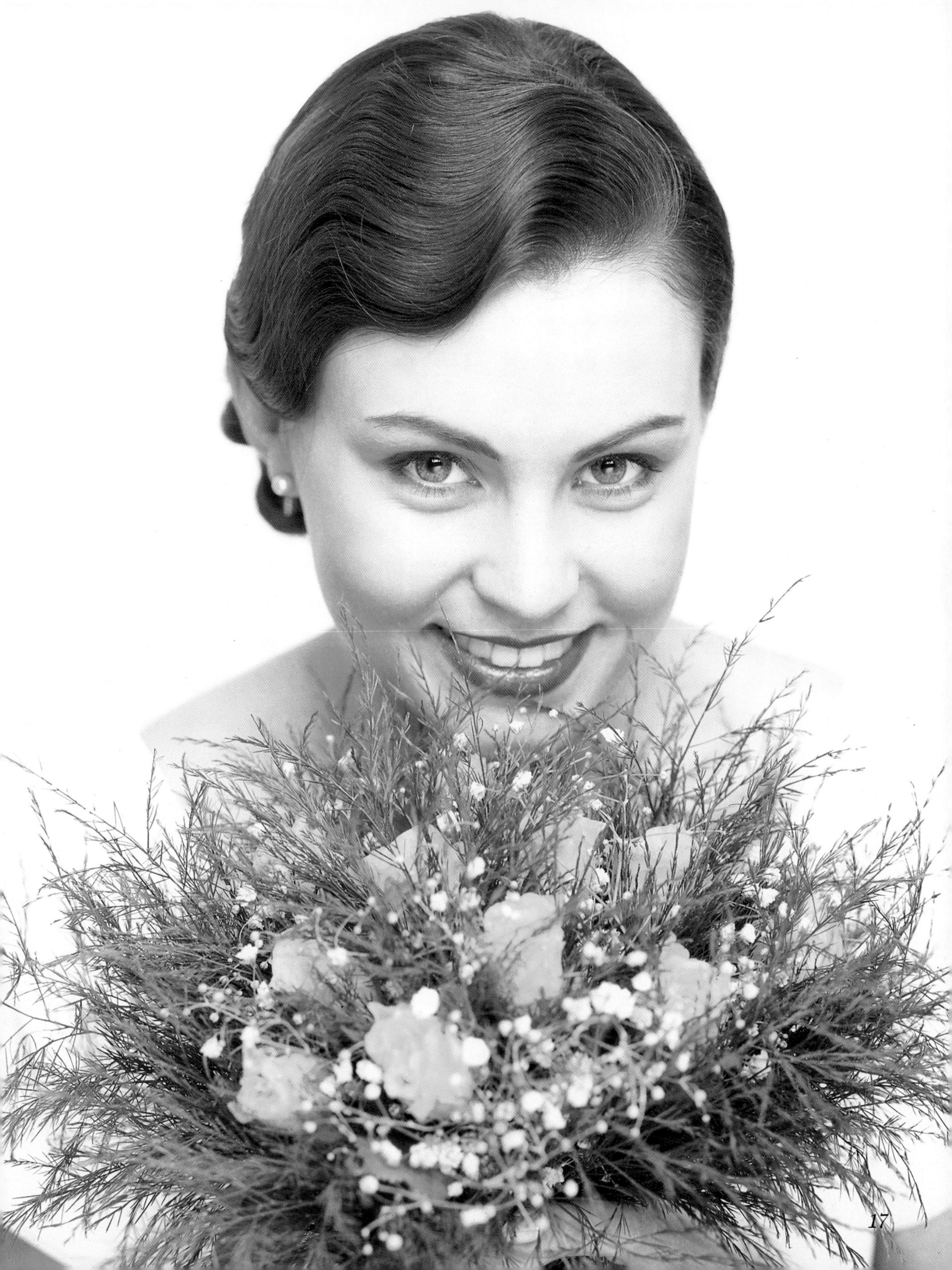

Accessories

aubles and beads add that finishing touch and make any bride sparkle. Traditional pearls and diamonds are perfect for formal gowns but many contemporary brides wear modern accessories that feature splashes of colour. Short or slim gowns with very little detailing provide the perfect canvas for a dazzling choker or a necklace, while more ornate gowns look better with a single item such as a drop pearl or a solitaire diamond.

Jewellery from a selection at Classics Bridal Hire Collection and Virgin Bride
Opposite Gloves: Classics Bridal Hire Collection

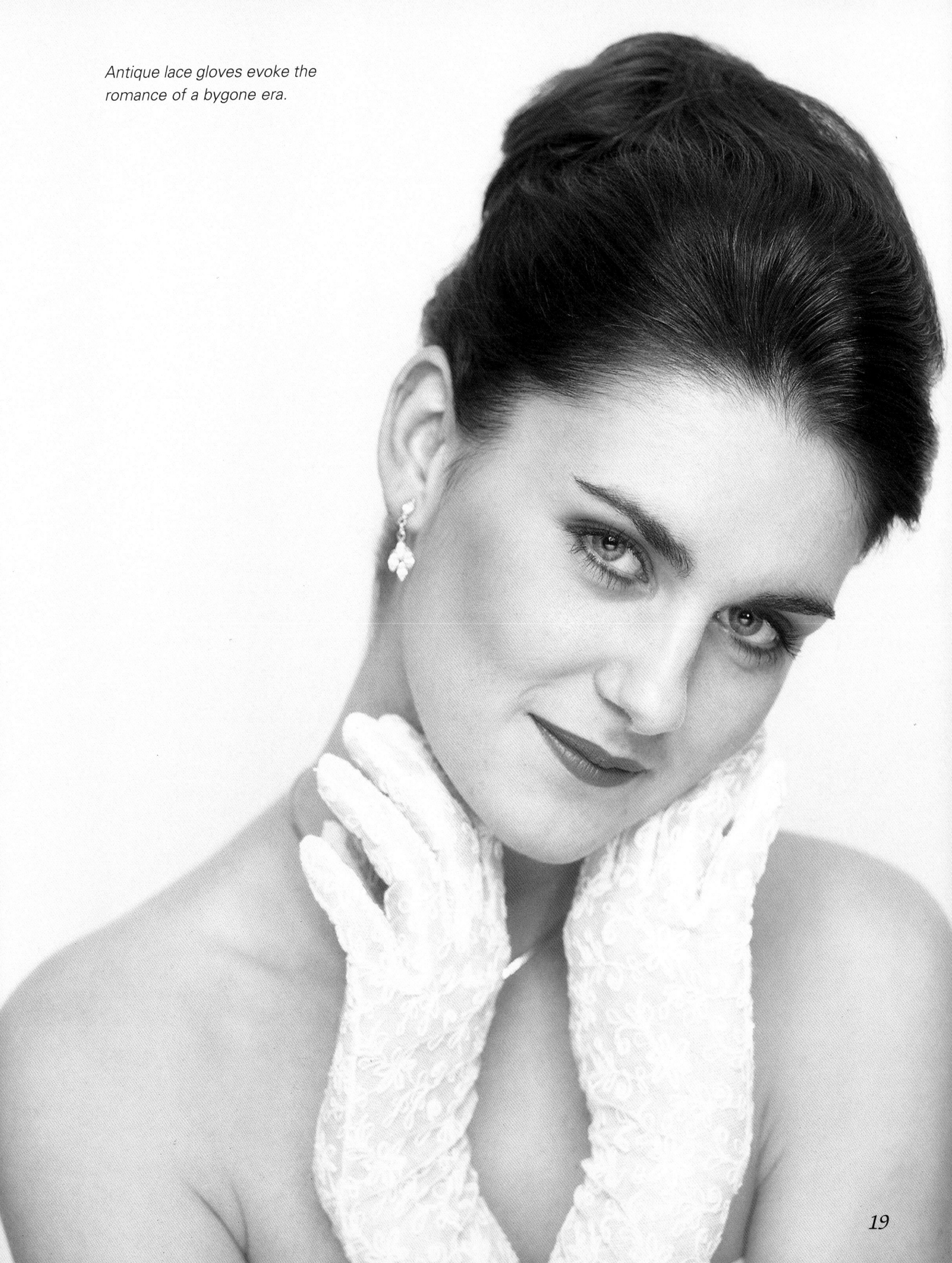

Antique lace gloves evoke the romance of a bygone era.

19

Dress rehearsal

Once all the ingredients for the bridal look have been chosen, it is essential to have a dress rehearsal, with the hairstyle, head-dress, tiara, veil and mock-up flowers in place. At this stage there is still time to make adjustments to ensure the look is perfect for the wedding day. It is also the time to ensure that the bride has remembered those little extras, such as a satin or embroidered bag to hold make-up essentials, a garter trimmed with blue ribbon, and something treasured to borrow from a special friend.

Traditional wedding slippers are made in silk or satin to match the dress, but as fabric doesn't give like leather, half a size bigger than normal is a good idea. Heels shouldn't be too high and the shoes should be worn indoors a few times prior to the wedding day to break them in and make sure they are comfortable. The style of the shoe is also important and should be appropriate to the time of year. Whatever style is chosen, the shoes should be worn at the final dress fitting to ensure the length is correct. If they have price stickers on the soles, this is the time to remove them.

Parasol, bag, shoes: Cocoa
Garter: Virgin Bride
Pearls: Classics Bridal Hire Collection

Opposite Dress and head-dress: Cocoa

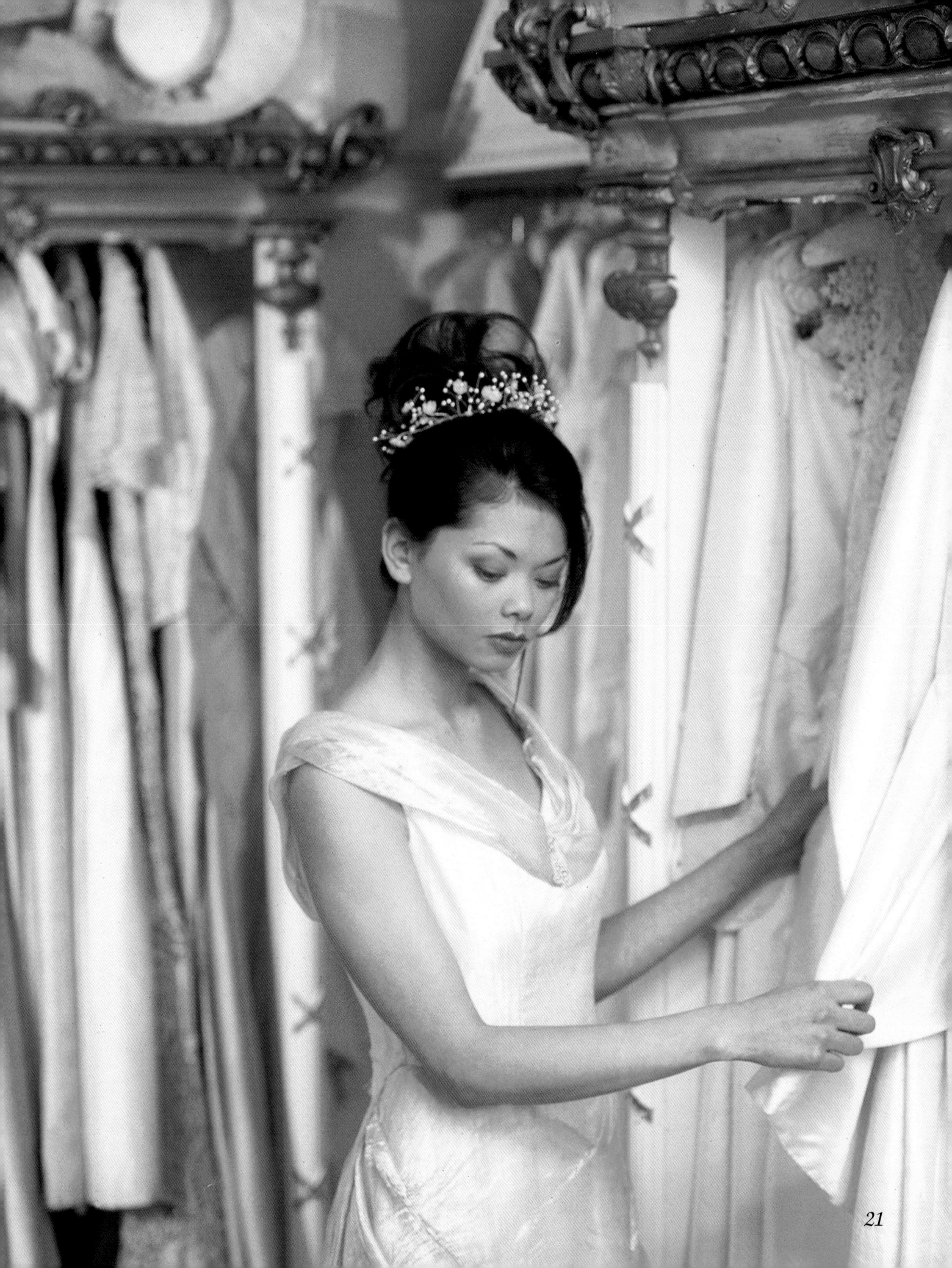

Bridesmaids

Young misses will love to have their hair blow-dried straight or tonged into soft curls. Floral tiaras should co-ordinate with the bride's bouquet and the overall colour theme.

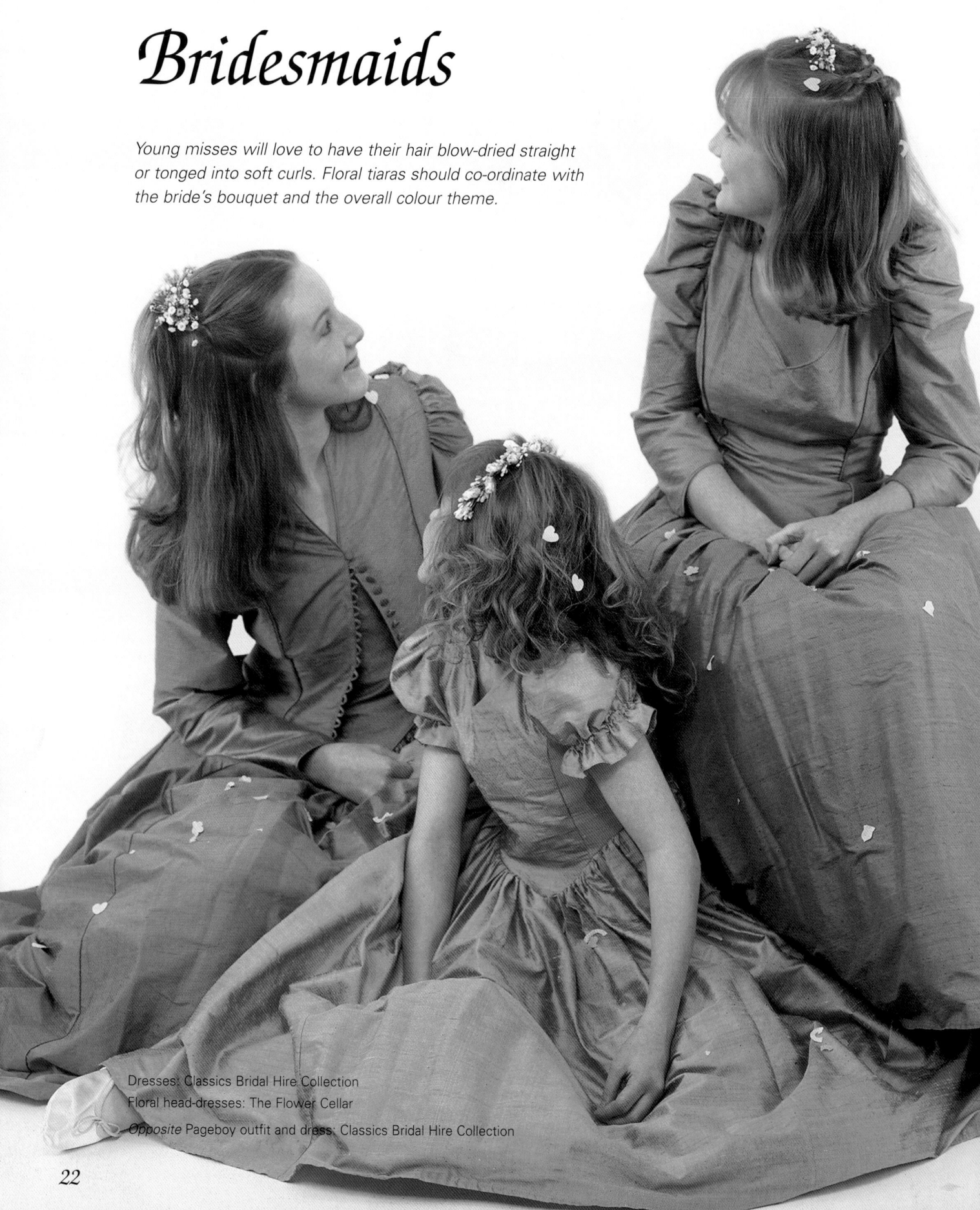

Dresses: Classics Bridal Hire Collection

Floral head-dresses: The Flower Cellar

Opposite Pageboy outfit and dress: Classics Bridal Hire Collection

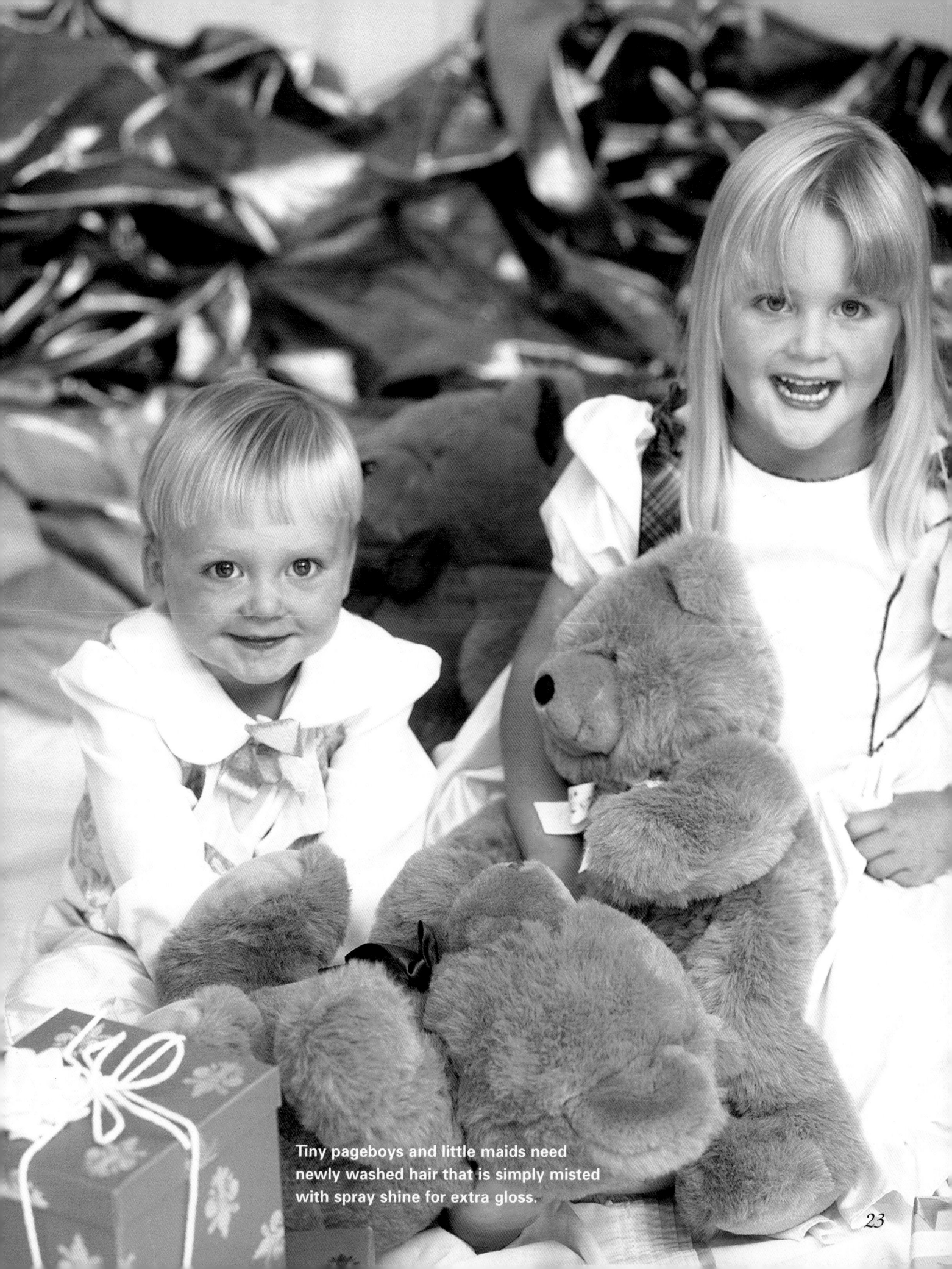

Tiny pageboys and little maids need
newly washed hair that is simply misted
with spray shine for extra gloss.

23

Maids of honour

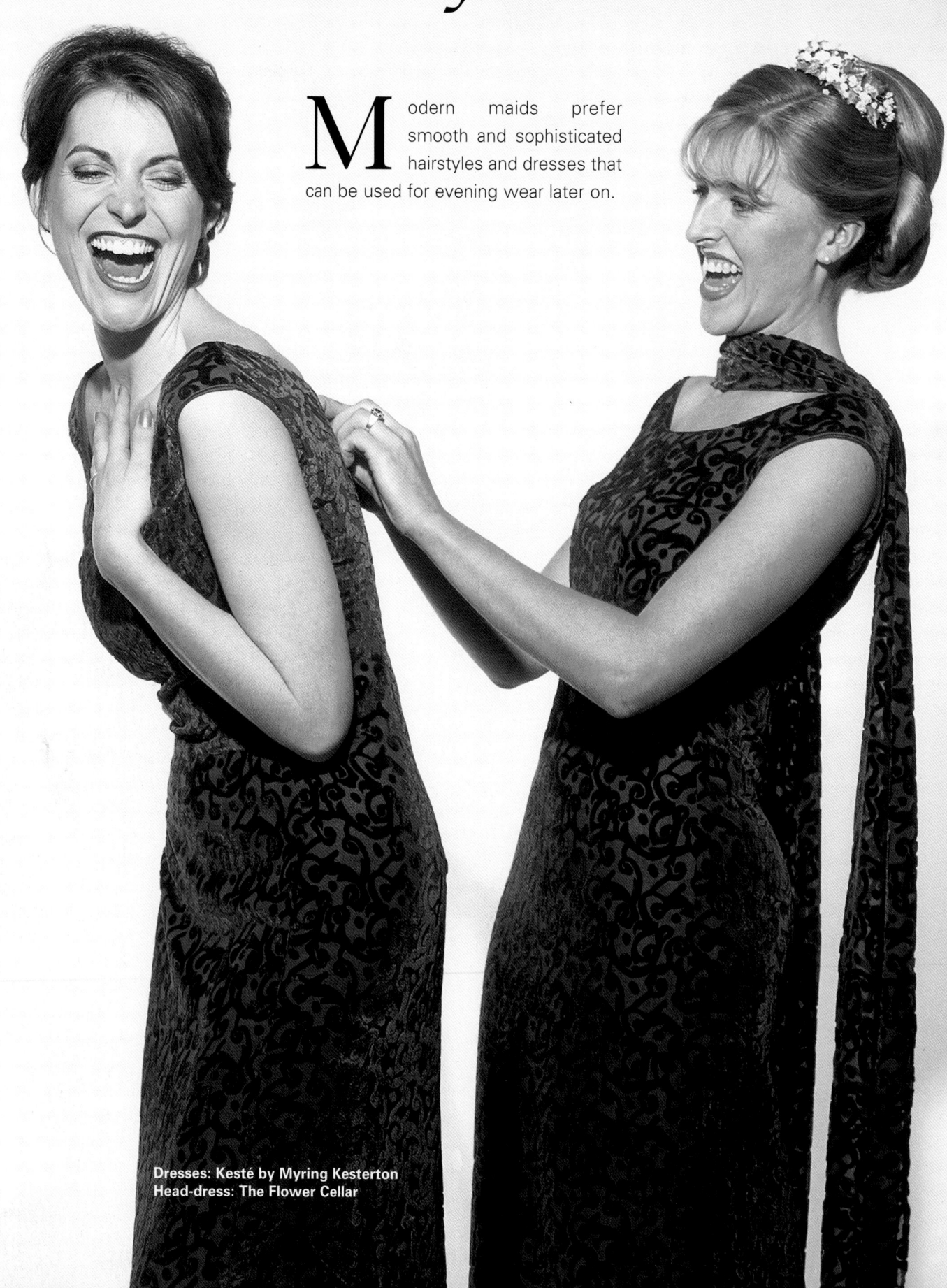

Modern maids prefer smooth and sophisticated hairstyles and dresses that can be used for evening wear later on.

Dresses: Kesté by Myring Kesterton
Head-dress: The Flower Cellar

Bride's mother & bridegroom

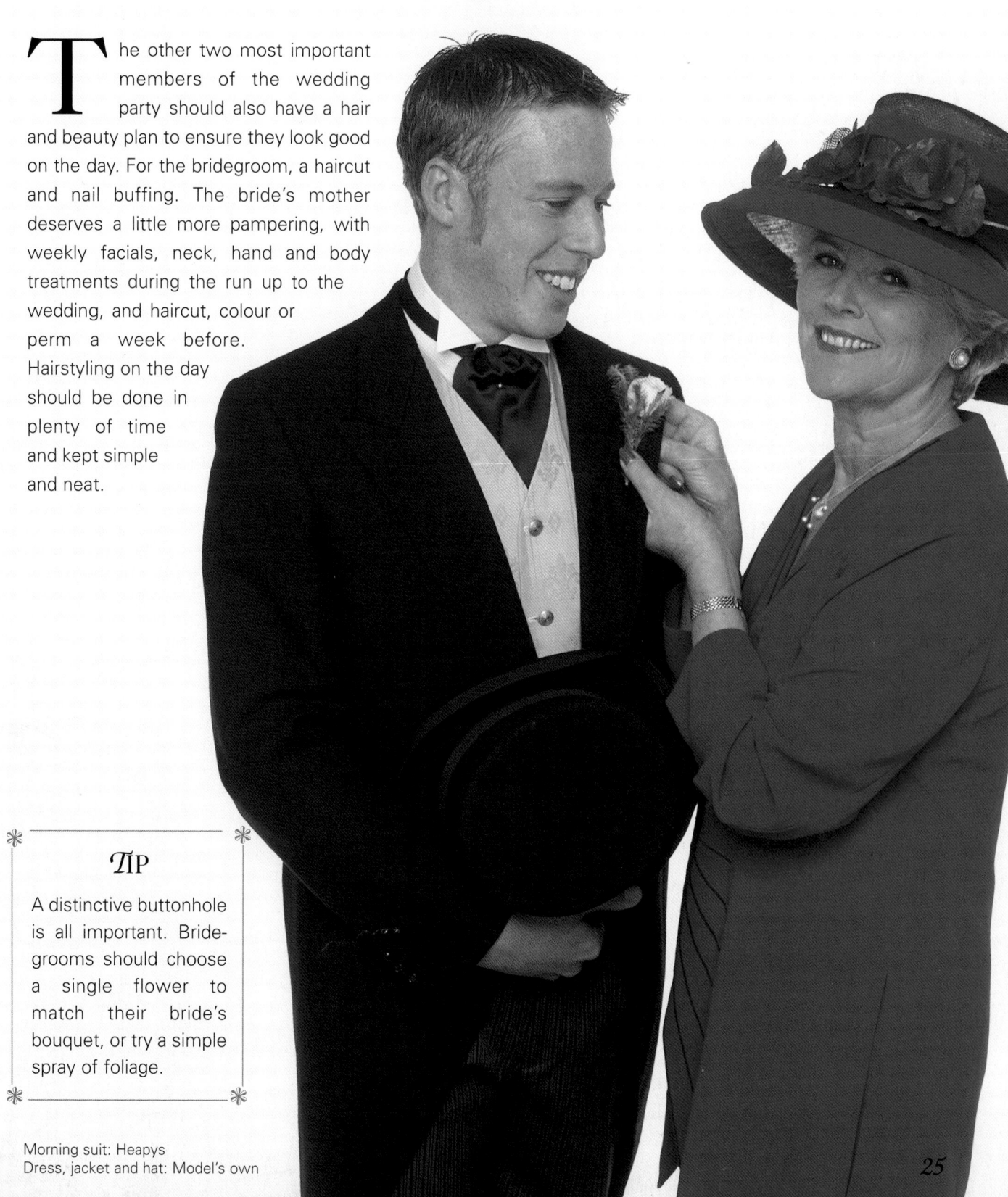

The other two most important members of the wedding party should also have a hair and beauty plan to ensure they look good on the day. For the bridegroom, a haircut and nail buffing. The bride's mother deserves a little more pampering, with weekly facials, neck, hand and body treatments during the run up to the wedding, and haircut, colour or perm a week before. Hairstyling on the day should be done in plenty of time and kept simple and neat.

Morning suit: Heapys
Dress, jacket and hat: Model's own

The big day

Soft, feminine bridal make-up is the order of the day. Blemishes should be disguised by applying concealer with a small brush, then liquid foundation to match the skin tone applied with a damp sponge. Start with a light covering and build up if necessary to give a flawless finish that will last all day. Set foundation by using a pad of cotton wool to press loose powder over the face and neck, then remove excess using downward strokes of a large powder brush. Blusher should be applied with a large brush to cheekbones and blended so it fades naturally towards hairline. Eyelids should be powdered to give a base, then softly coloured with the lightest of eyeshadows. Accentuate brows with a pencil and slick them into place with a tiny dab of hair gel. Lashes should be curled, then two thin coats of mascara applied. If lashes clog, gently separate with a small comb. Lips should be outlined in pencil and filled in using a lipbrush, then glossed over for a dewy finish.

The perfume the bride chooses will forever recall memories of her wedding day so it is important that she picks wisely. The key to finding the right fragrance is to identify the type of bride. A spring bride who chooses pale pink and peach colours with soft flowing fabrics, tiny garden flowers and ultra-feminine accessories will ruin the effect with a musk-based scent that is more suited to a glamorous evening reception or winter wedding. The romantic bride who wears reams of chiffon or antique lace and carries pastel roses or a wild-flower bouquet needs a gentle floral fragrance. The classic bride with her full veil, simple head-dress and full-skirted gown or corset dress needs a timeless fragrance with rose or lavender, while traditional brides can choose a heavier, more powerful scent. Wacky brides who wear colourful dresses can set the tone with a daring fragrance of amber and a twist of grapefruit, while the young bride should opt for the freshness of a water-based, lighter scent.

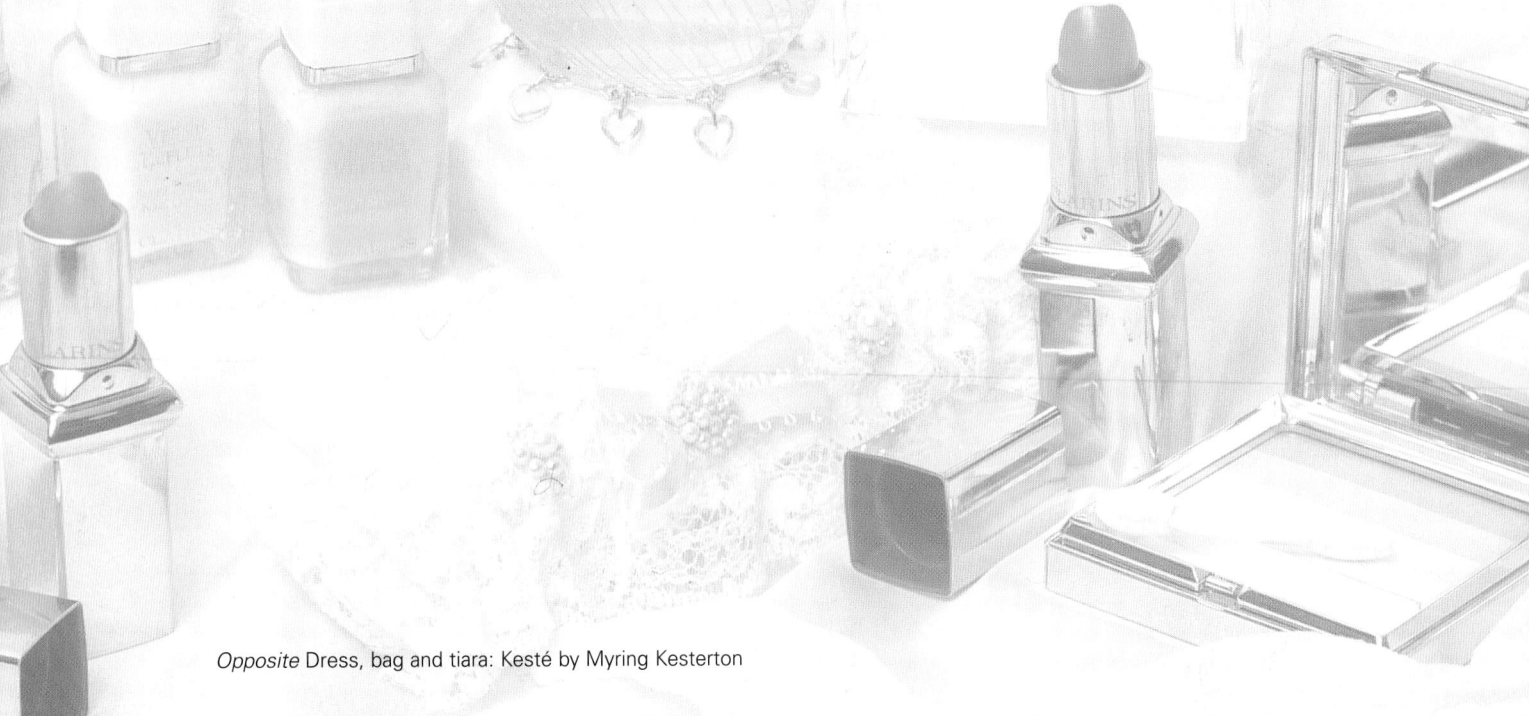

Opposite Dress, bag and tiara: Kesté by Myring Kesterton

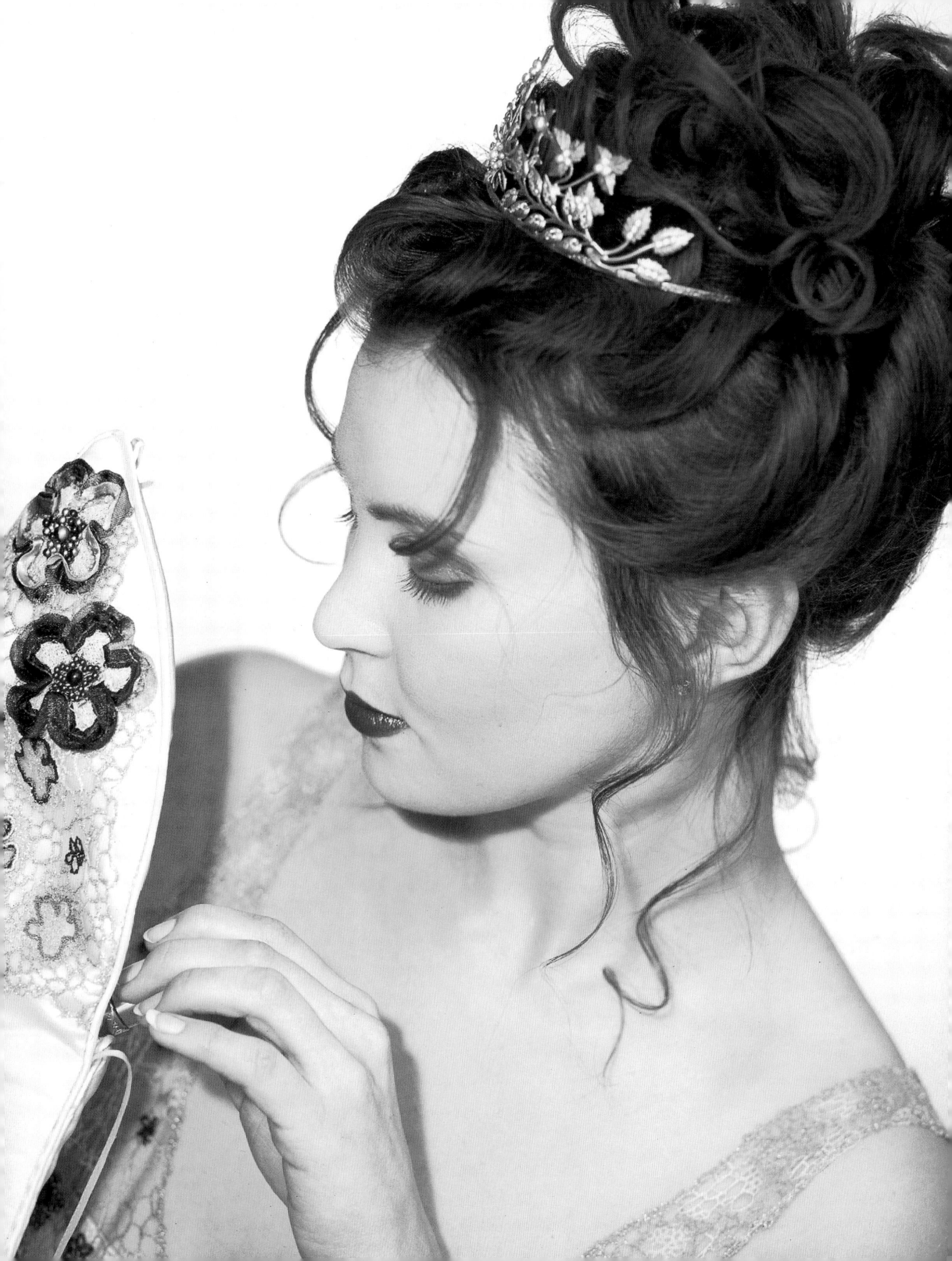

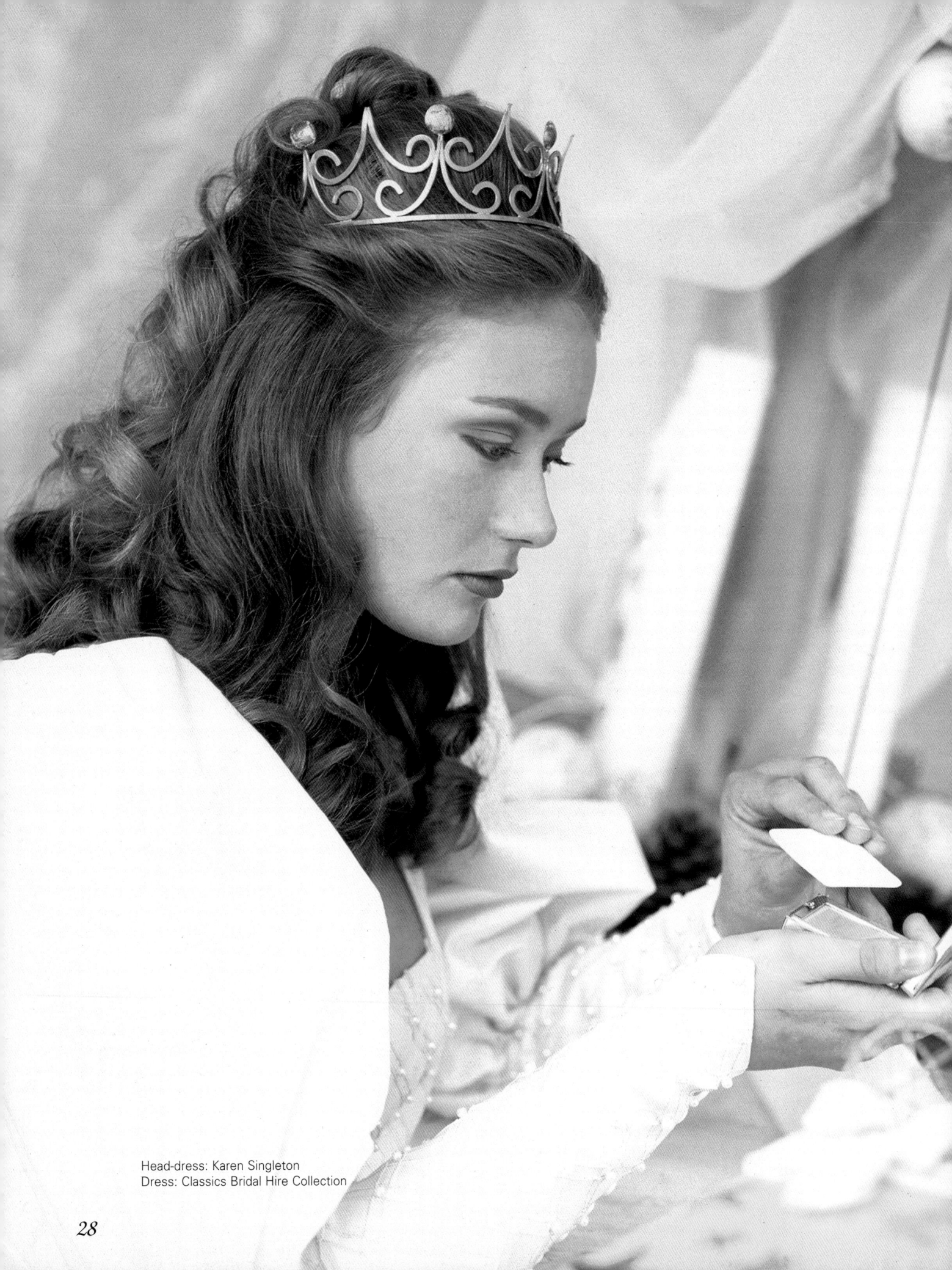

Head-dress: Karen Singleton
Dress: Classics Bridal Hire Collection

Bridal style gallery

34 romantic looks

Our beautiful bridal collection features 34 romantic wedding-day styles. Choose from classic, timeless looks or from alternative styles for the contemporary bride. Take inspiration from the basic shape and line but personalise the looks to suit individual hair type and texture.

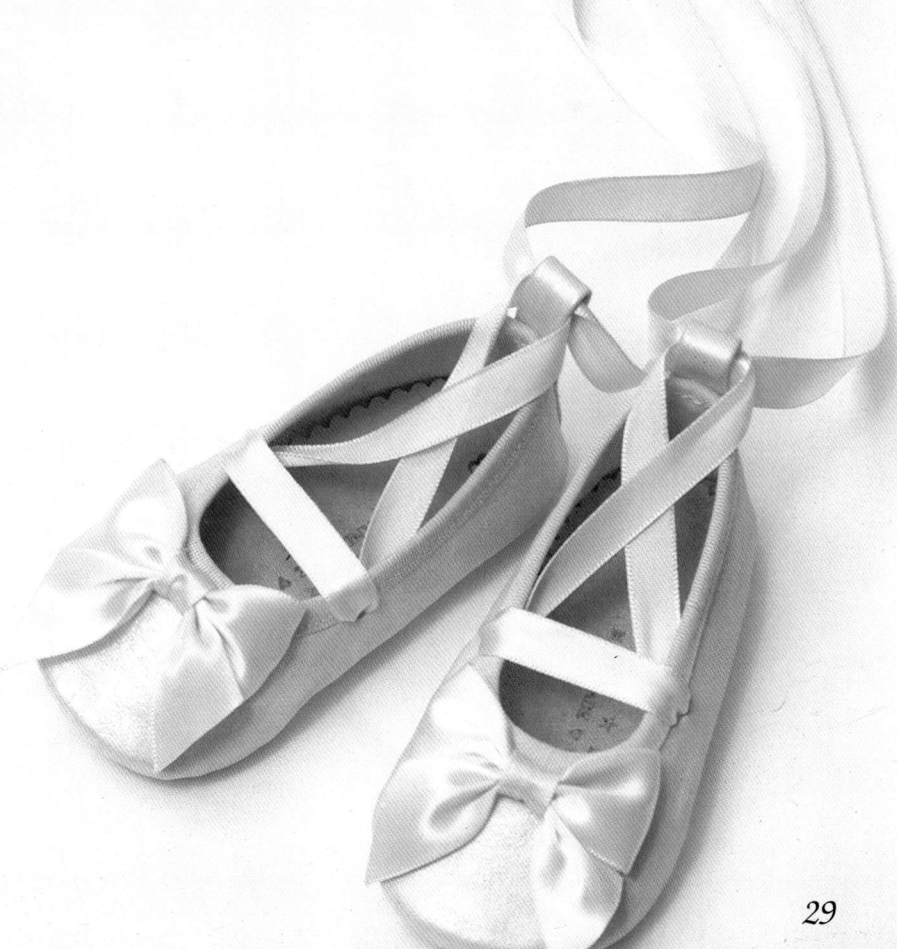

Ballet shoes: Cocoa

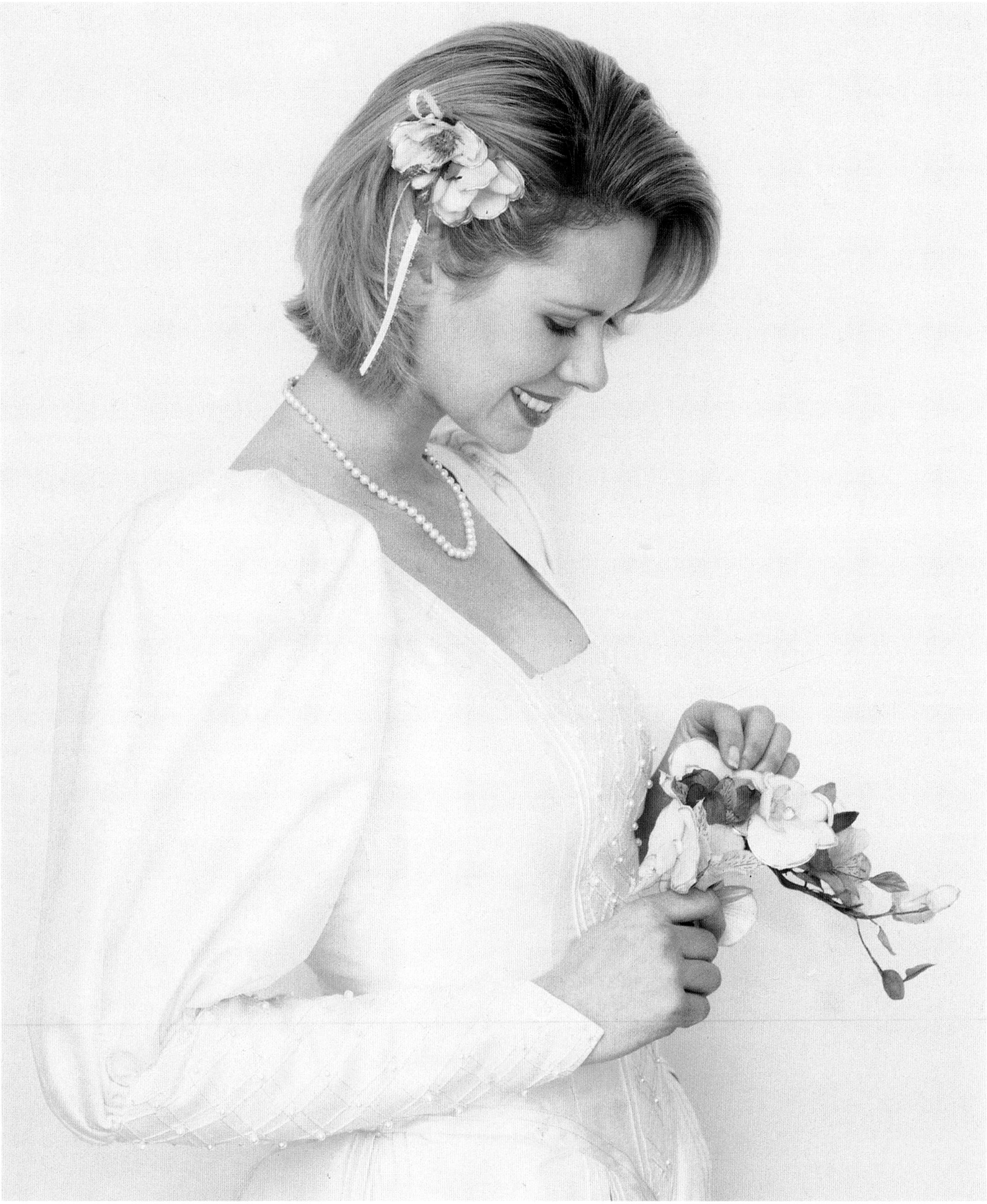

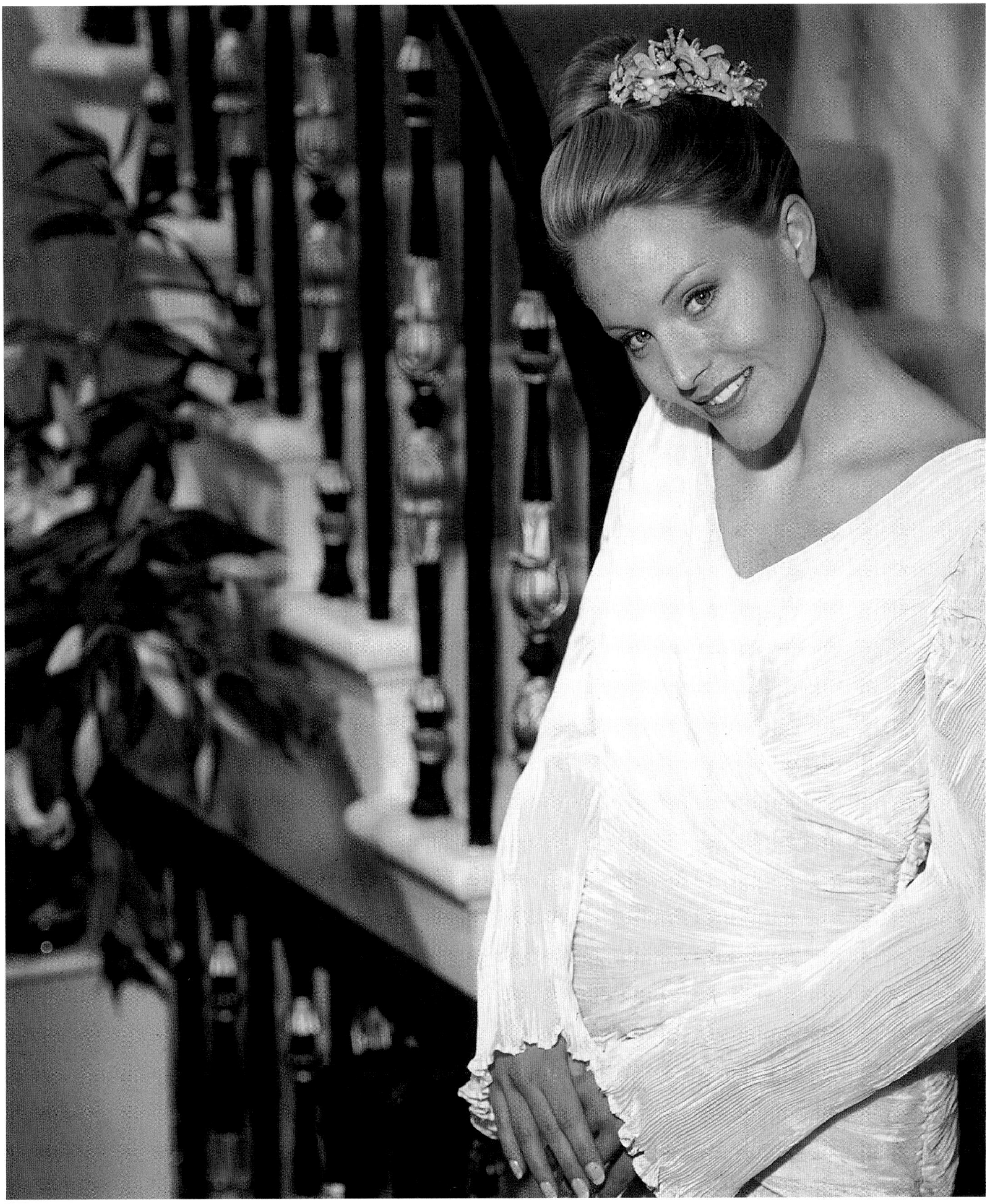

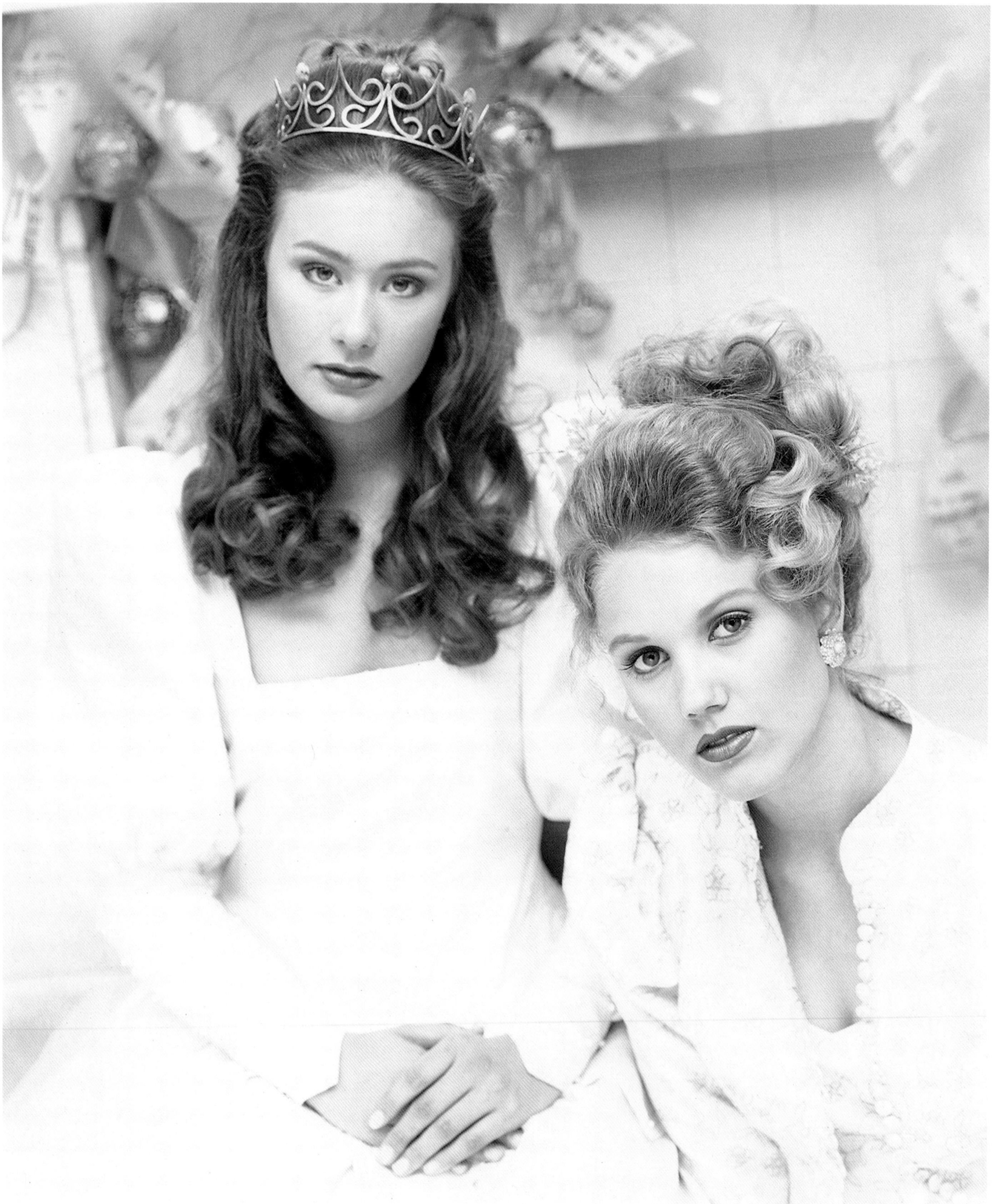

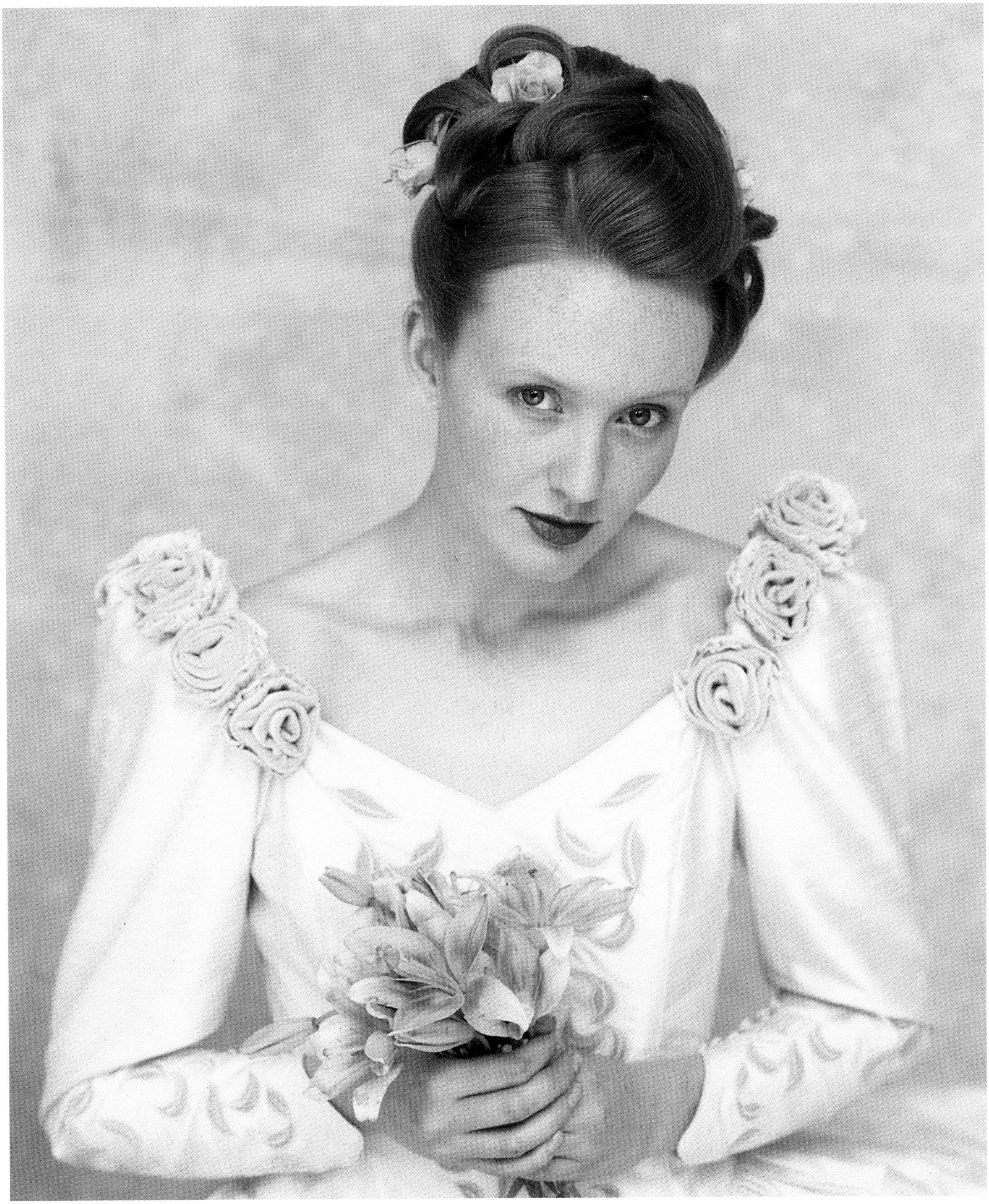

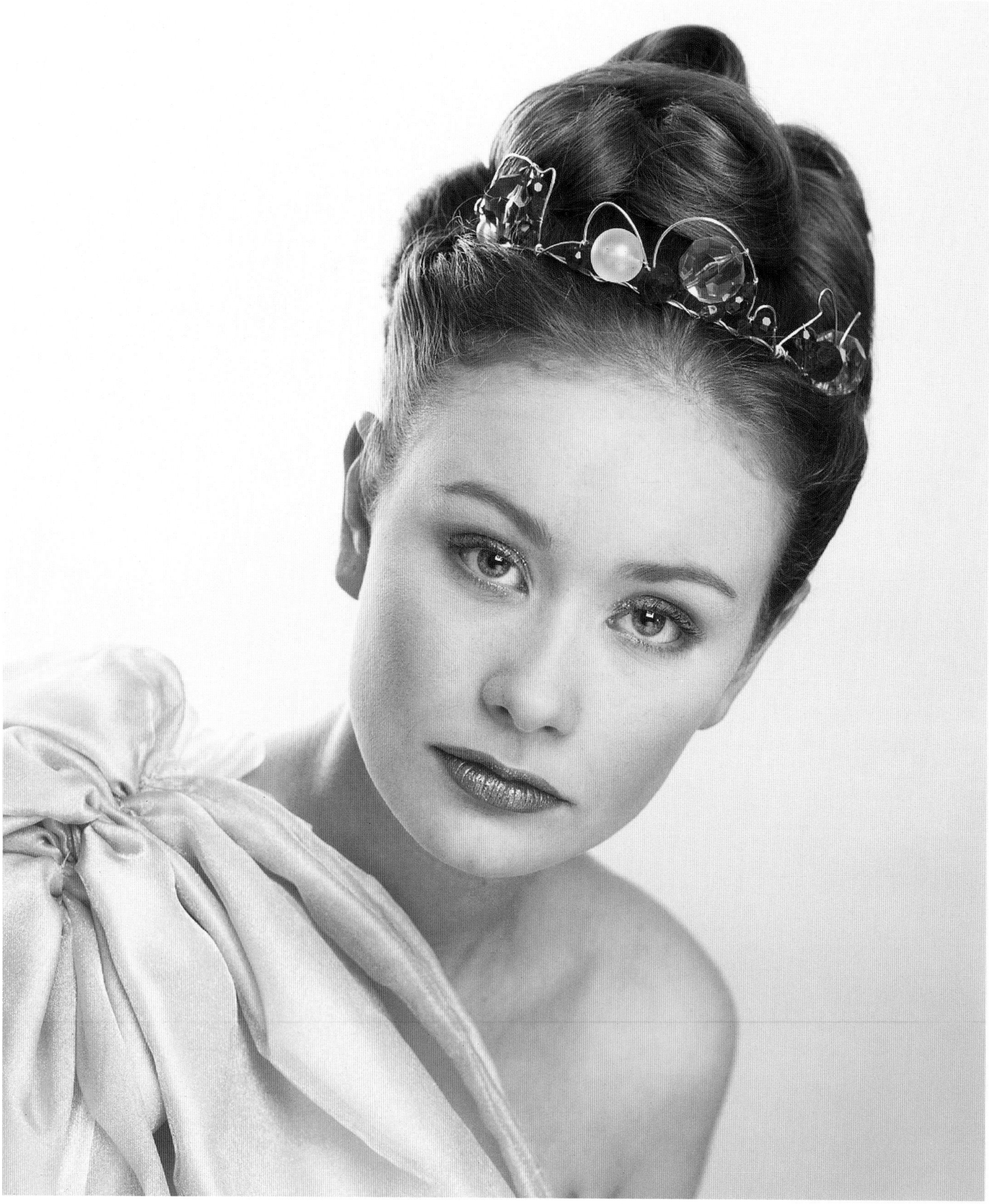

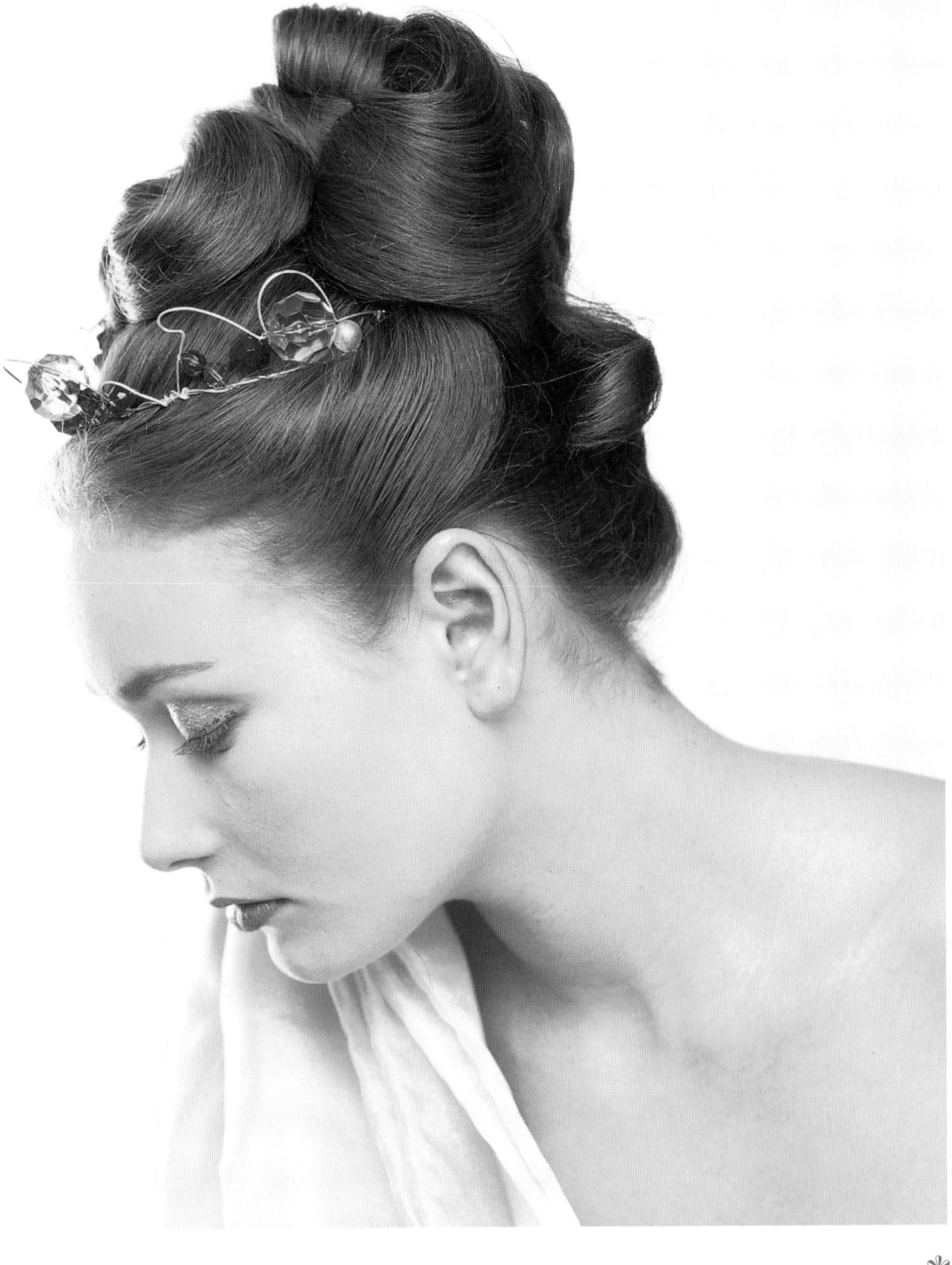

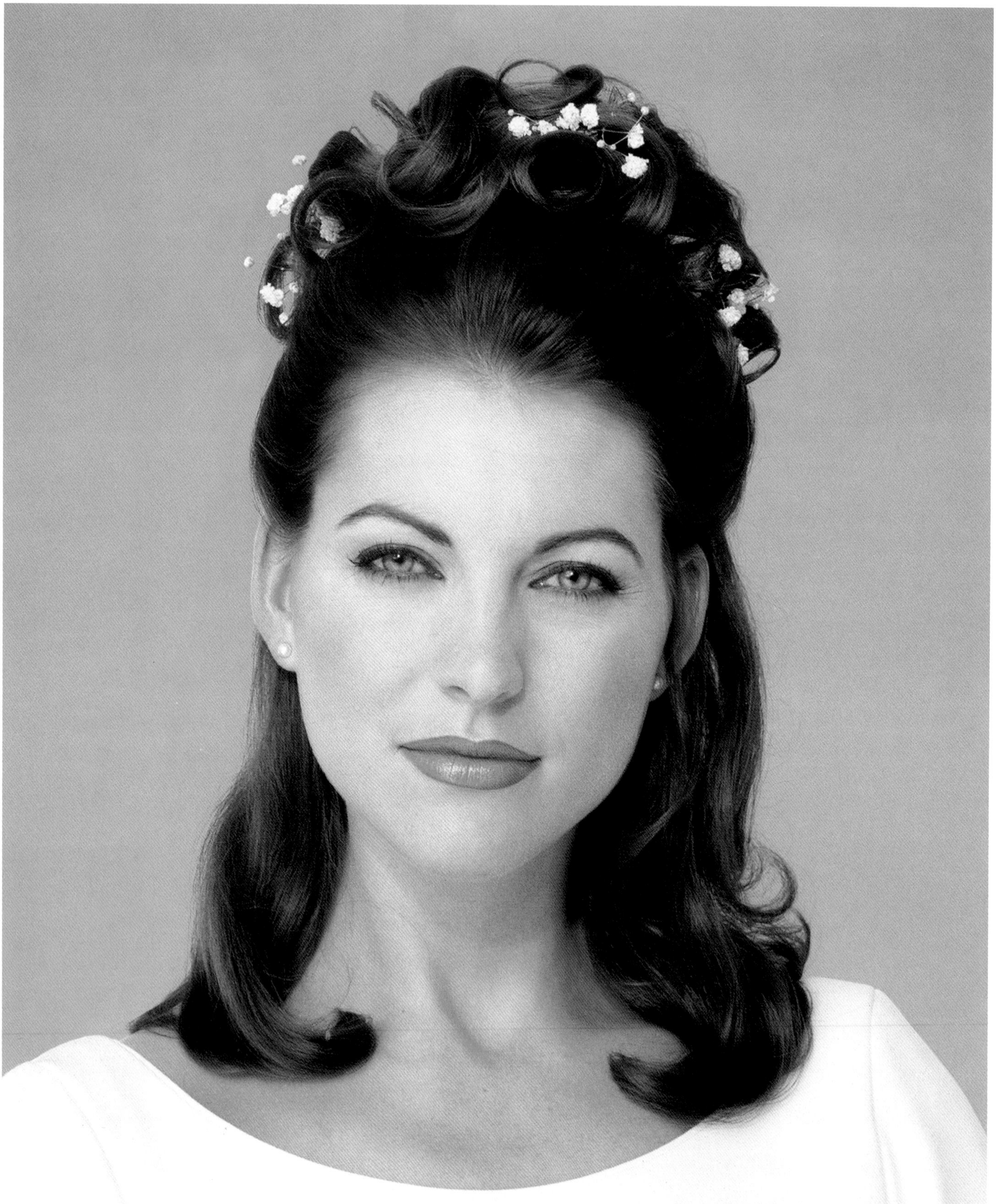

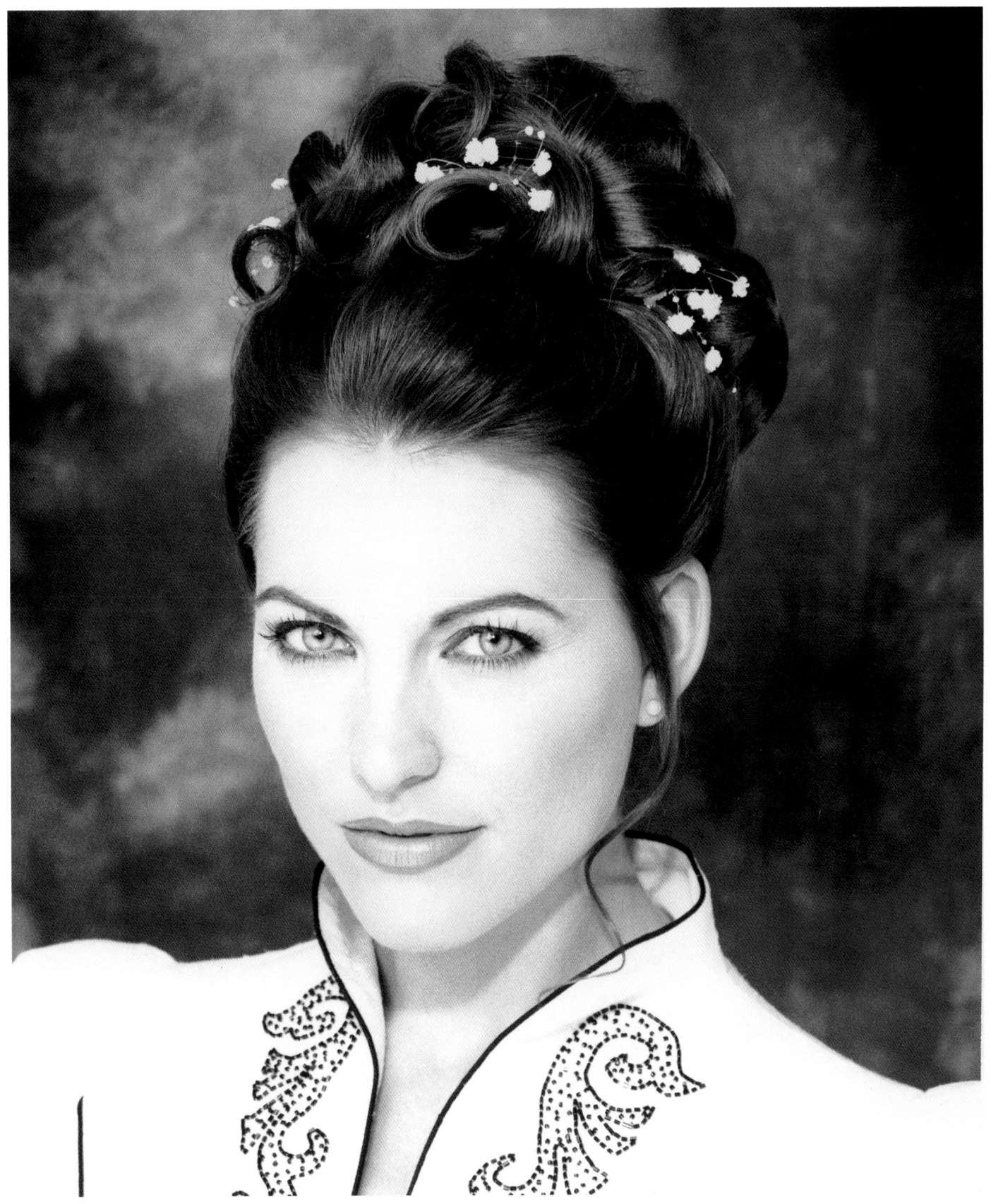

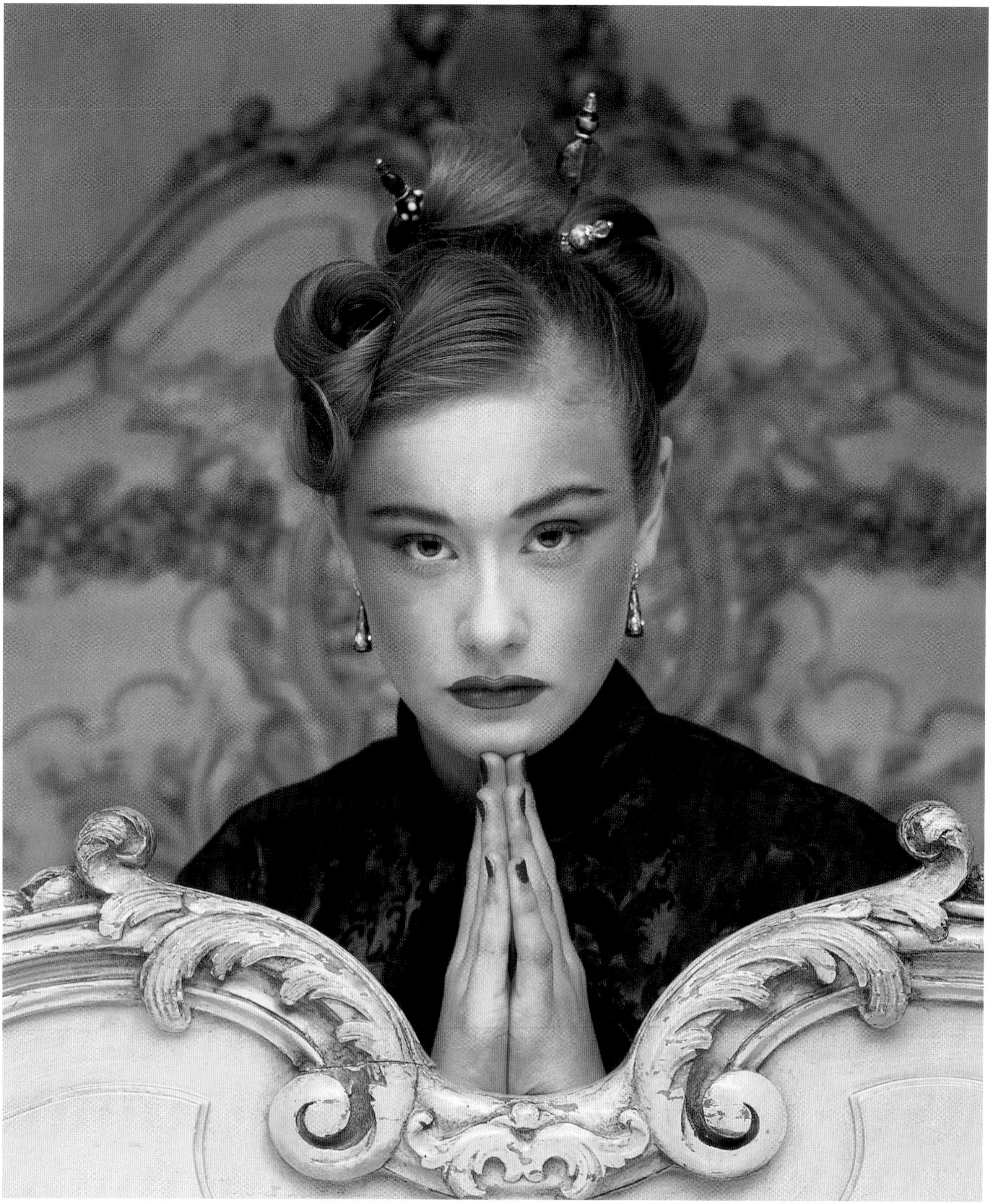

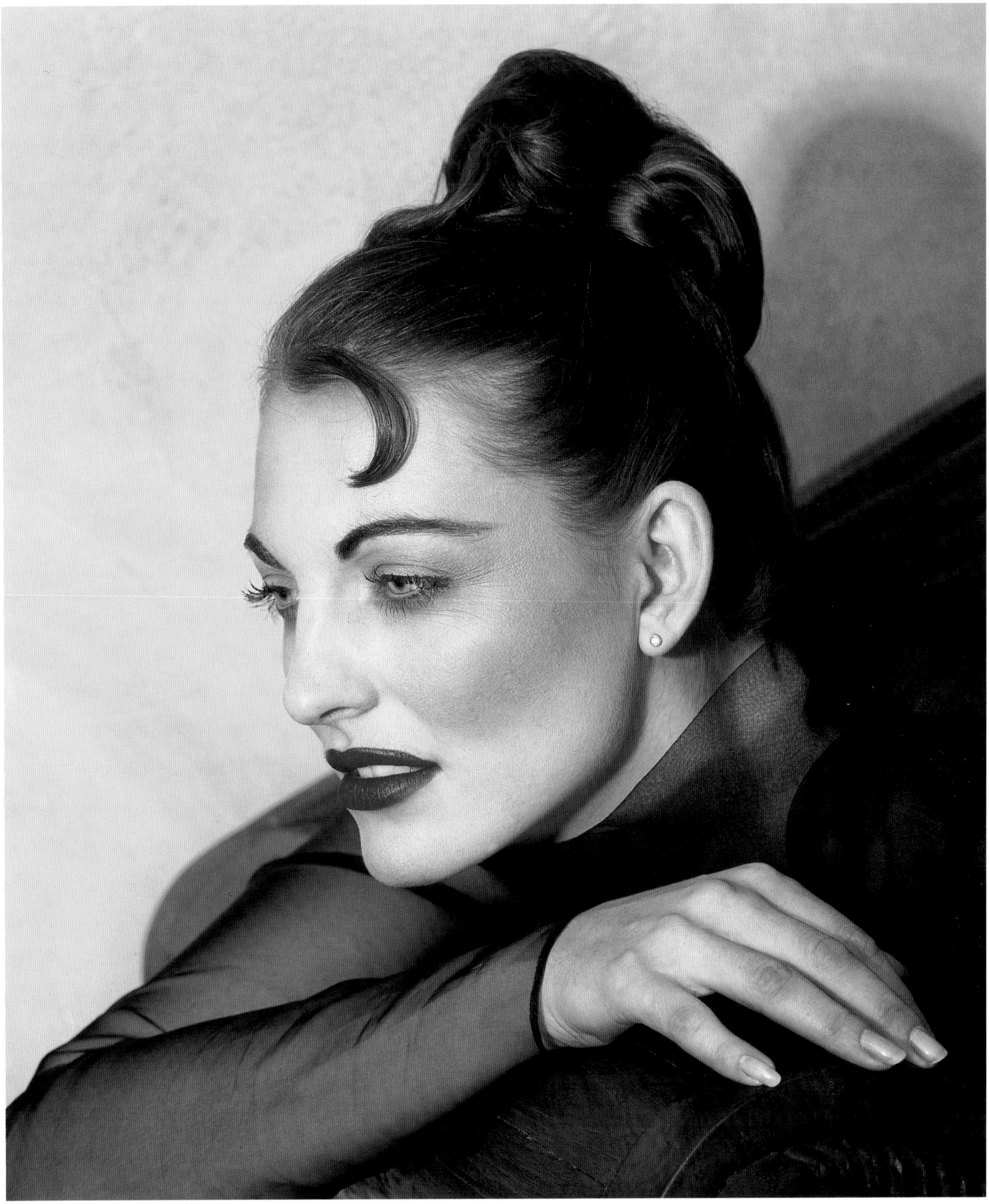

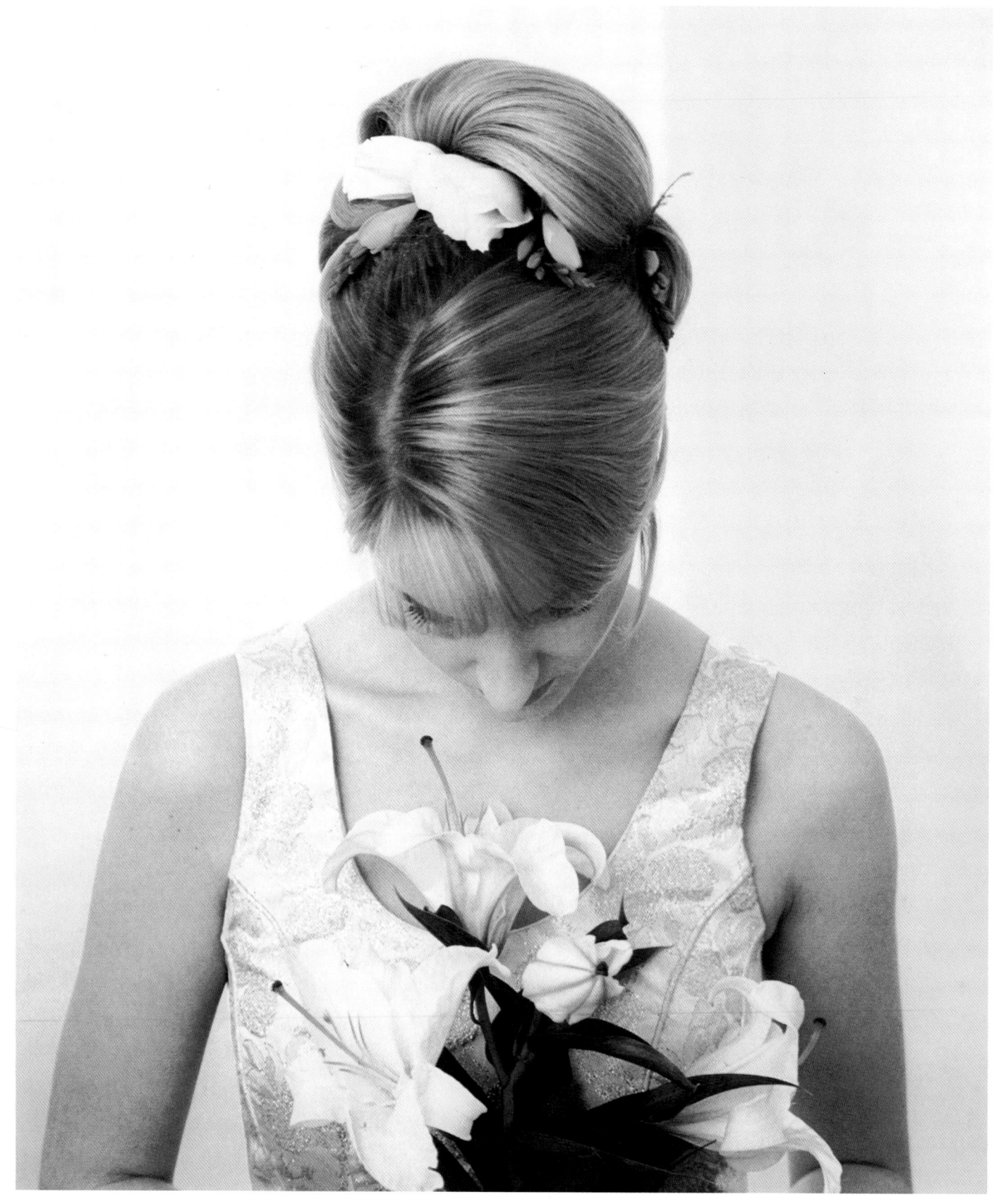

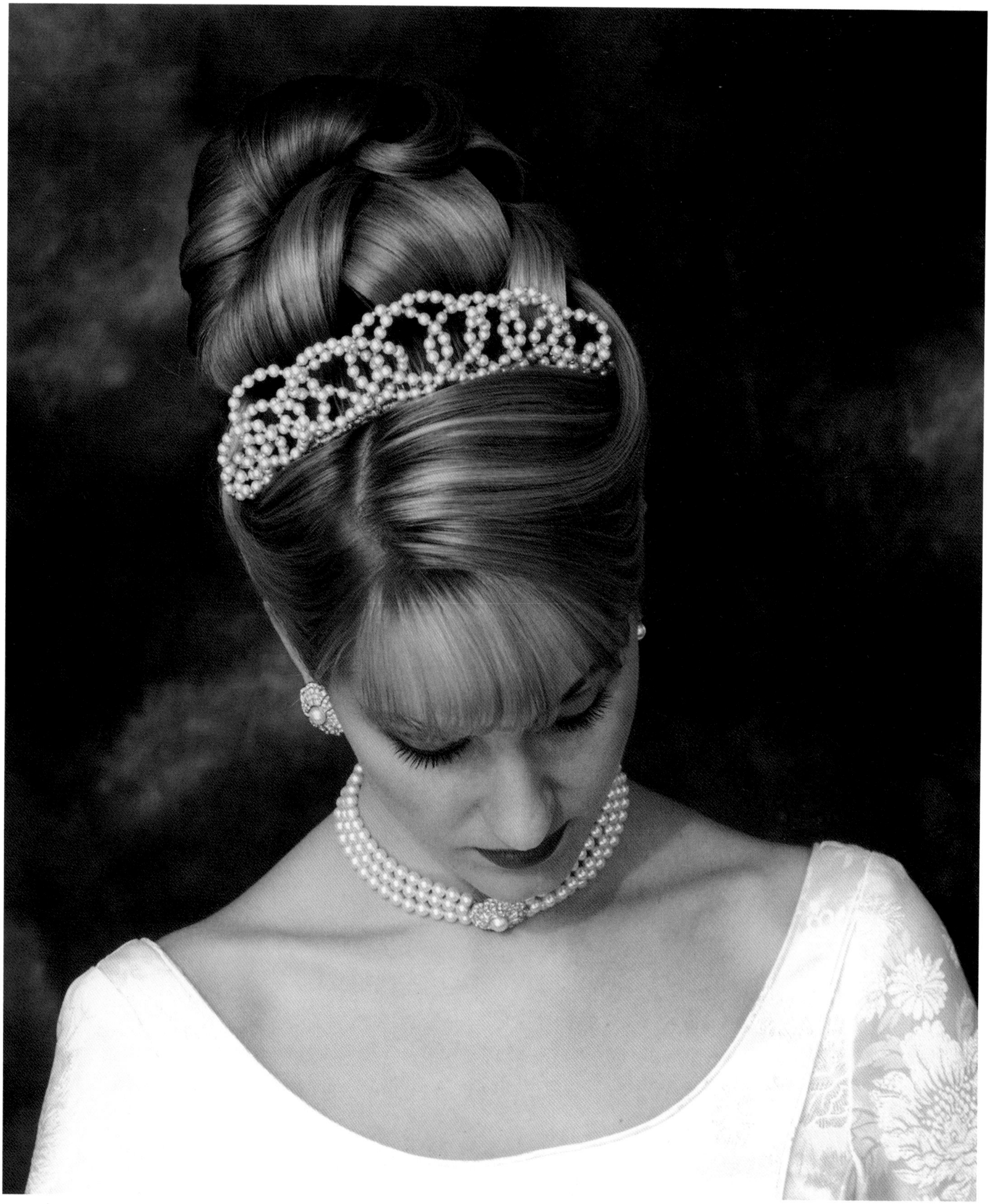

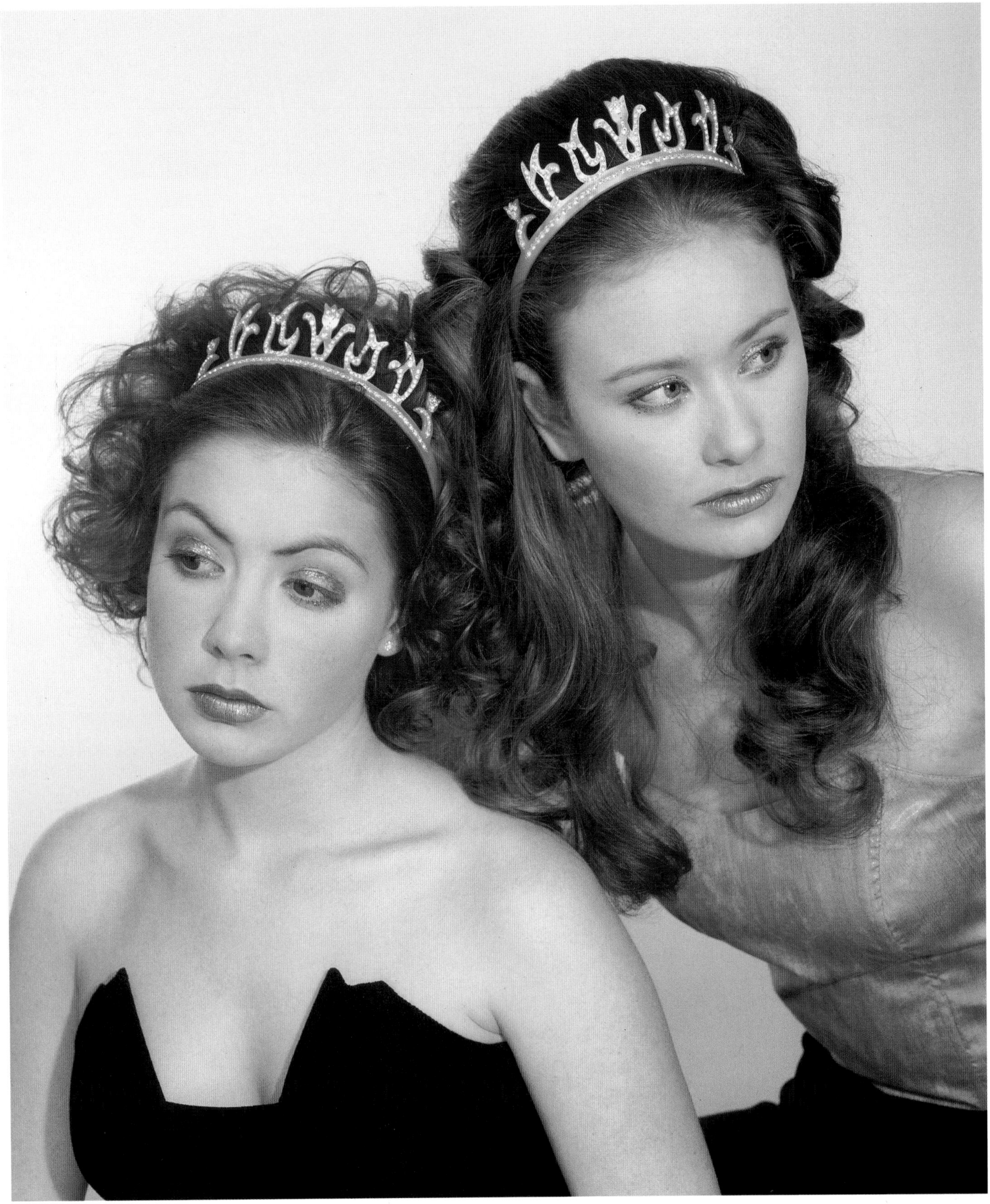

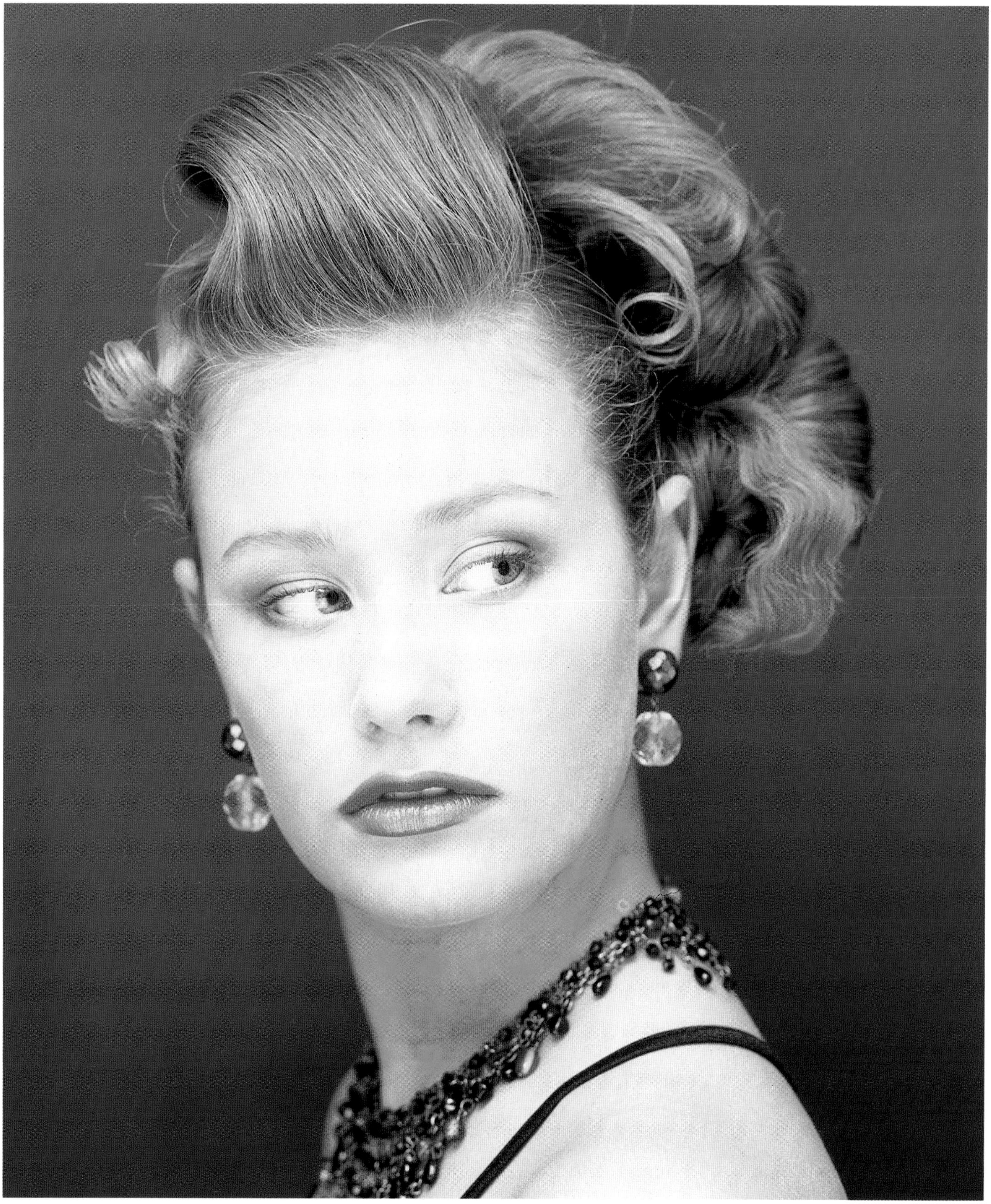

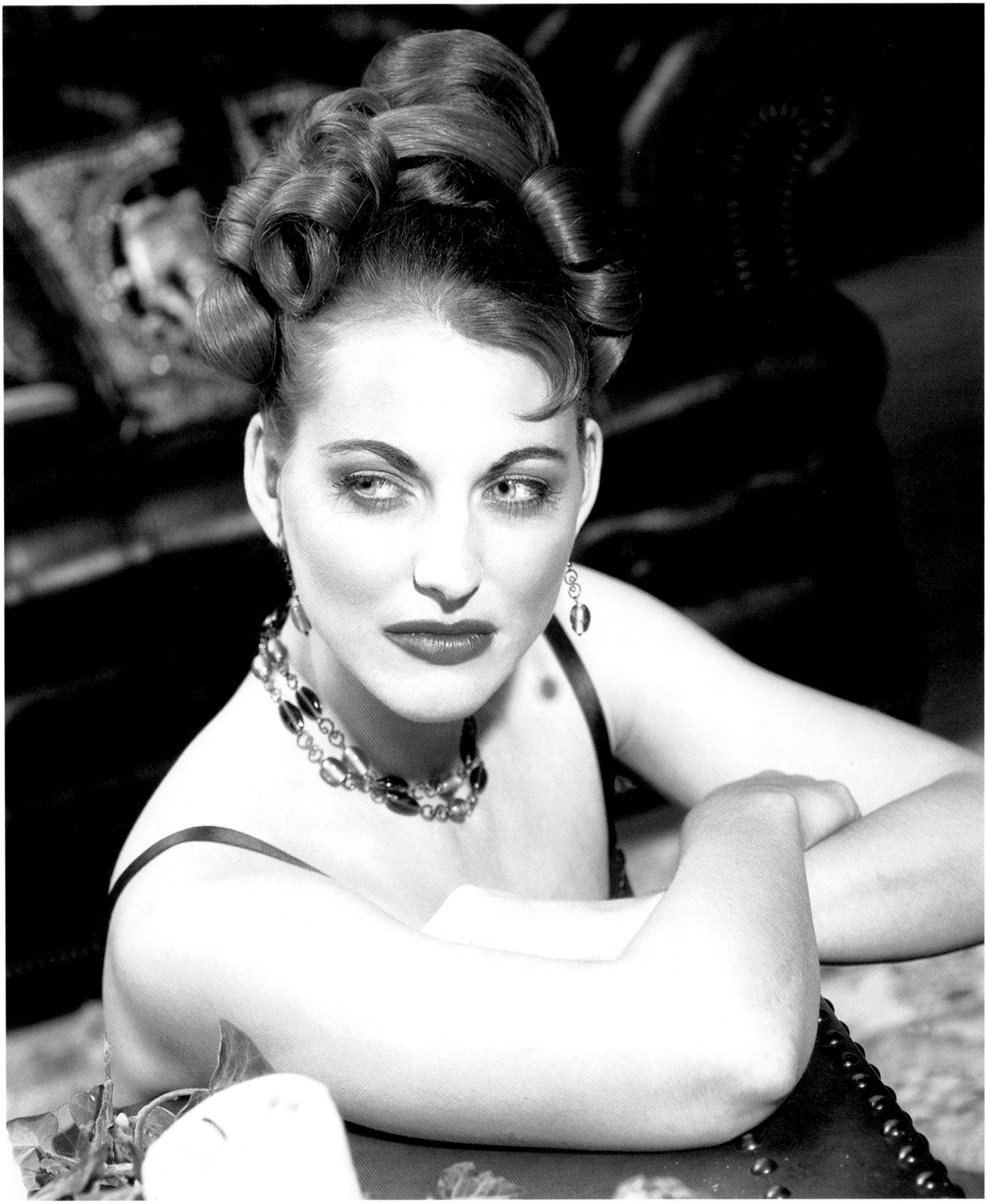

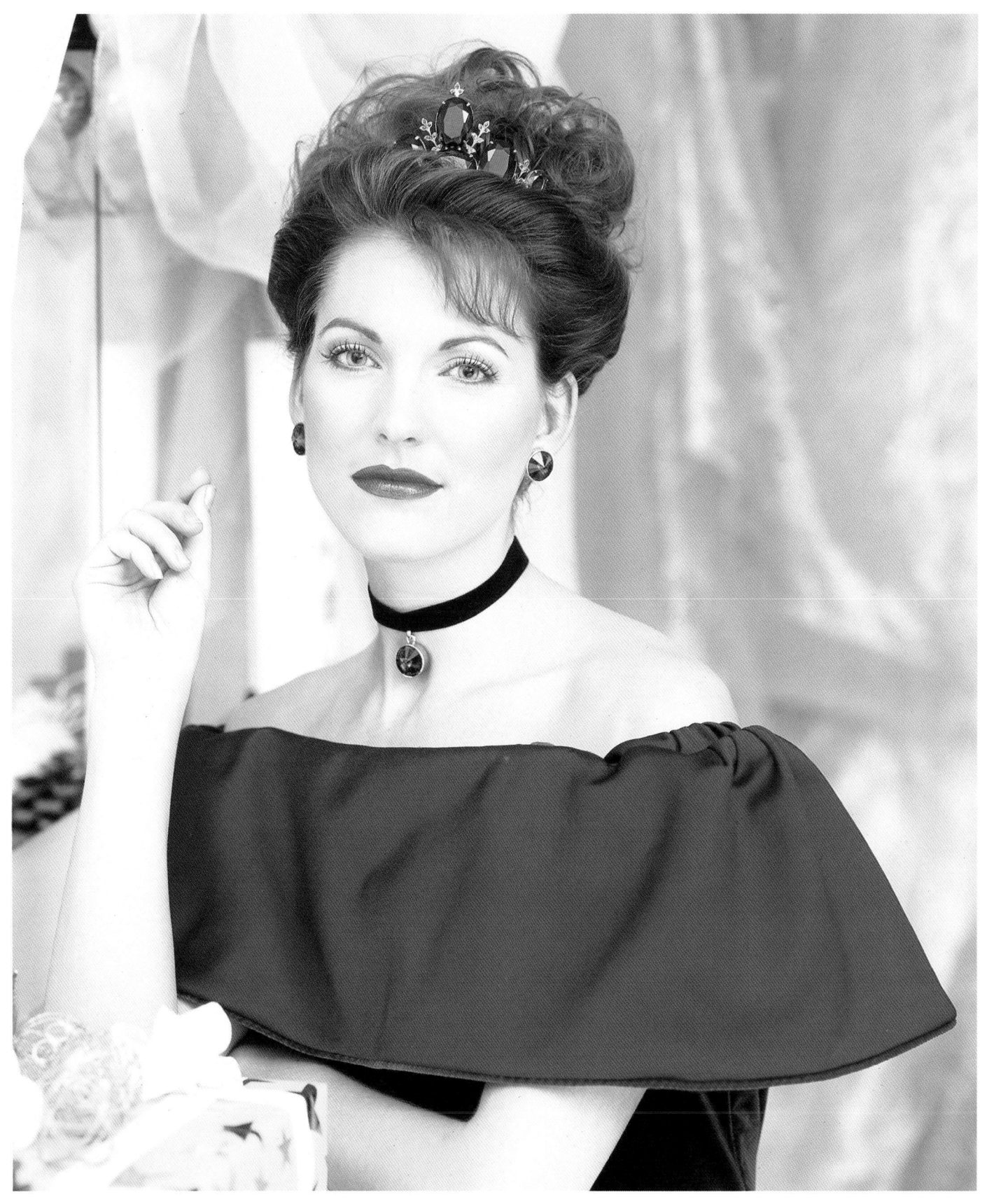

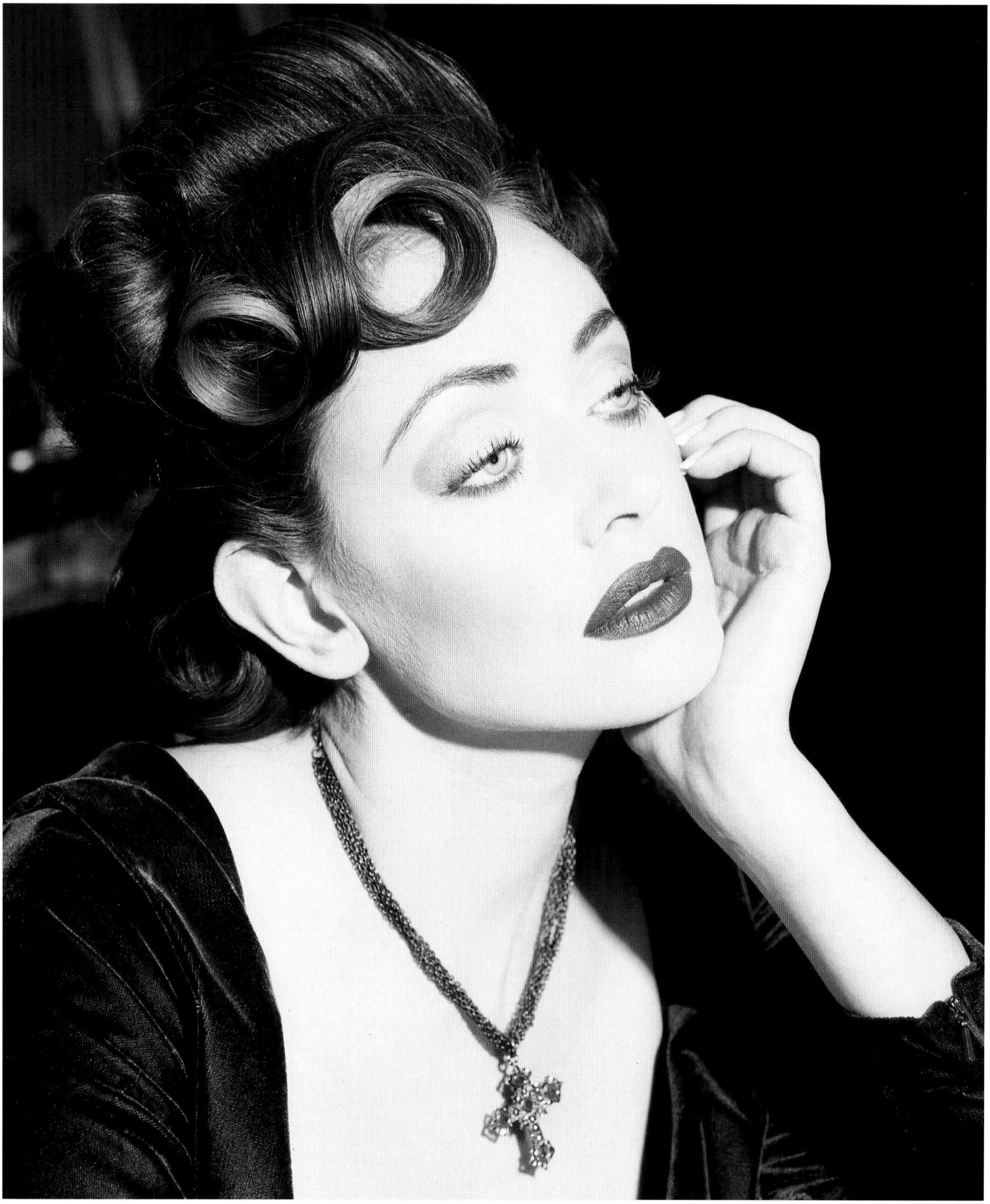

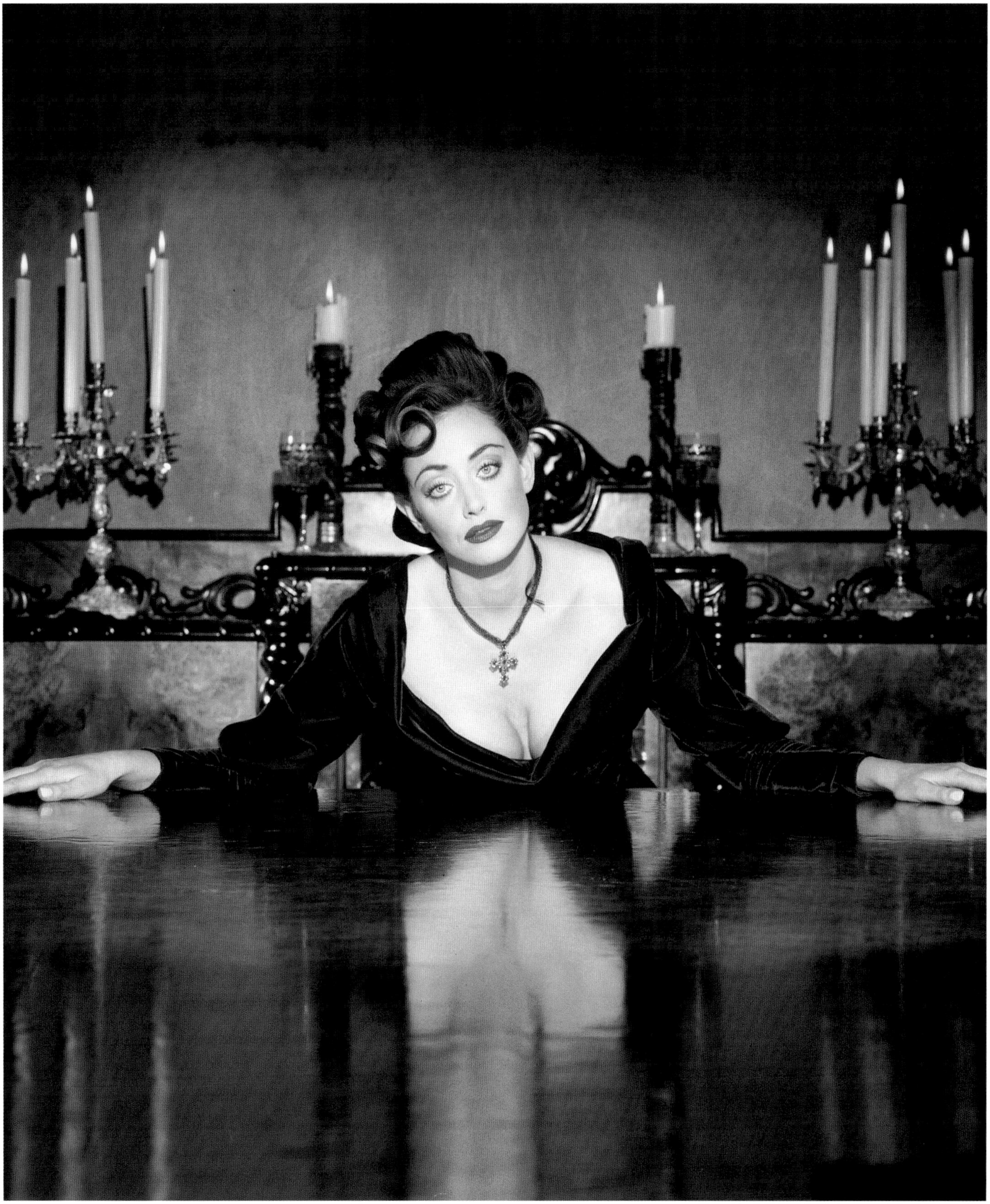

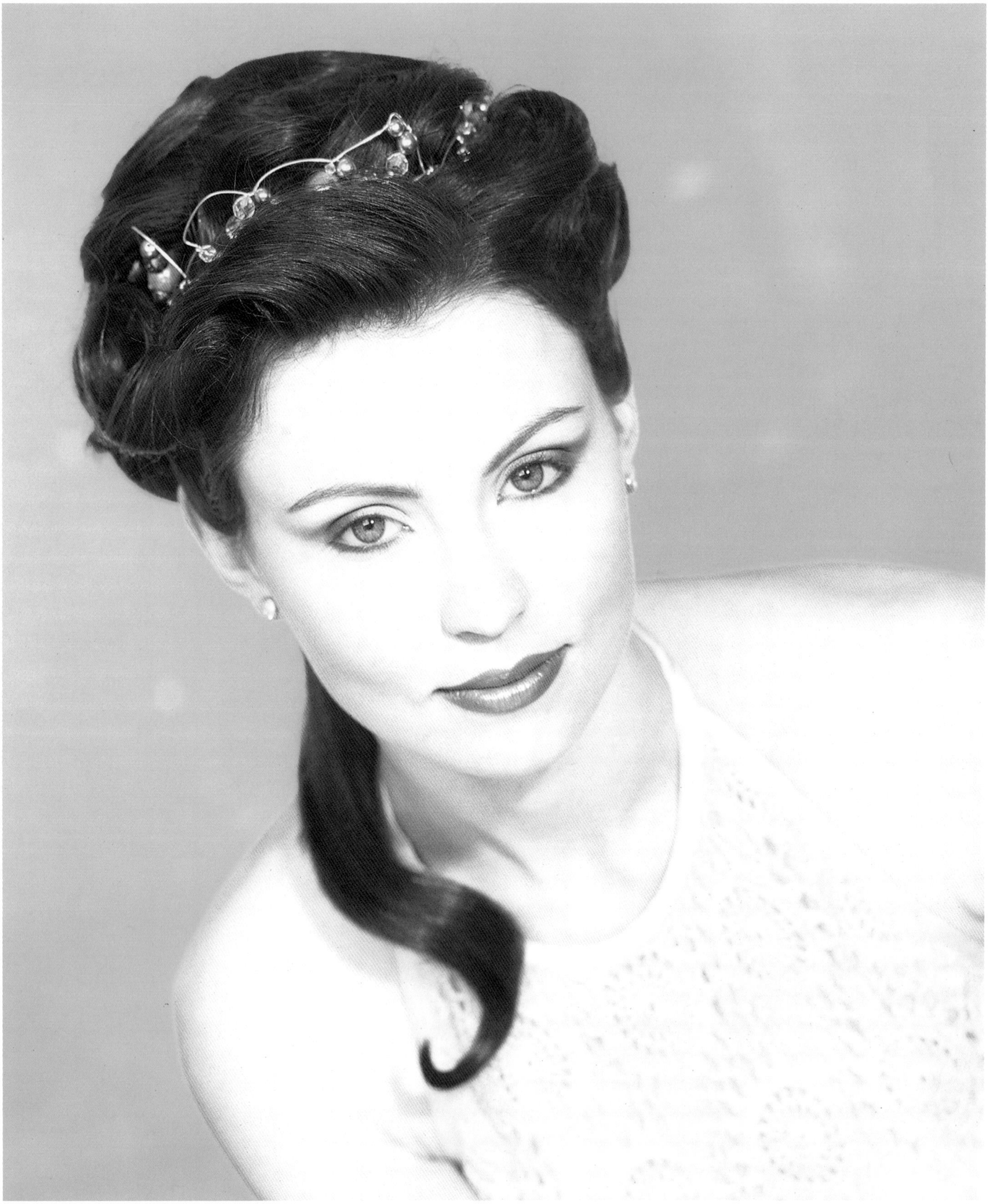

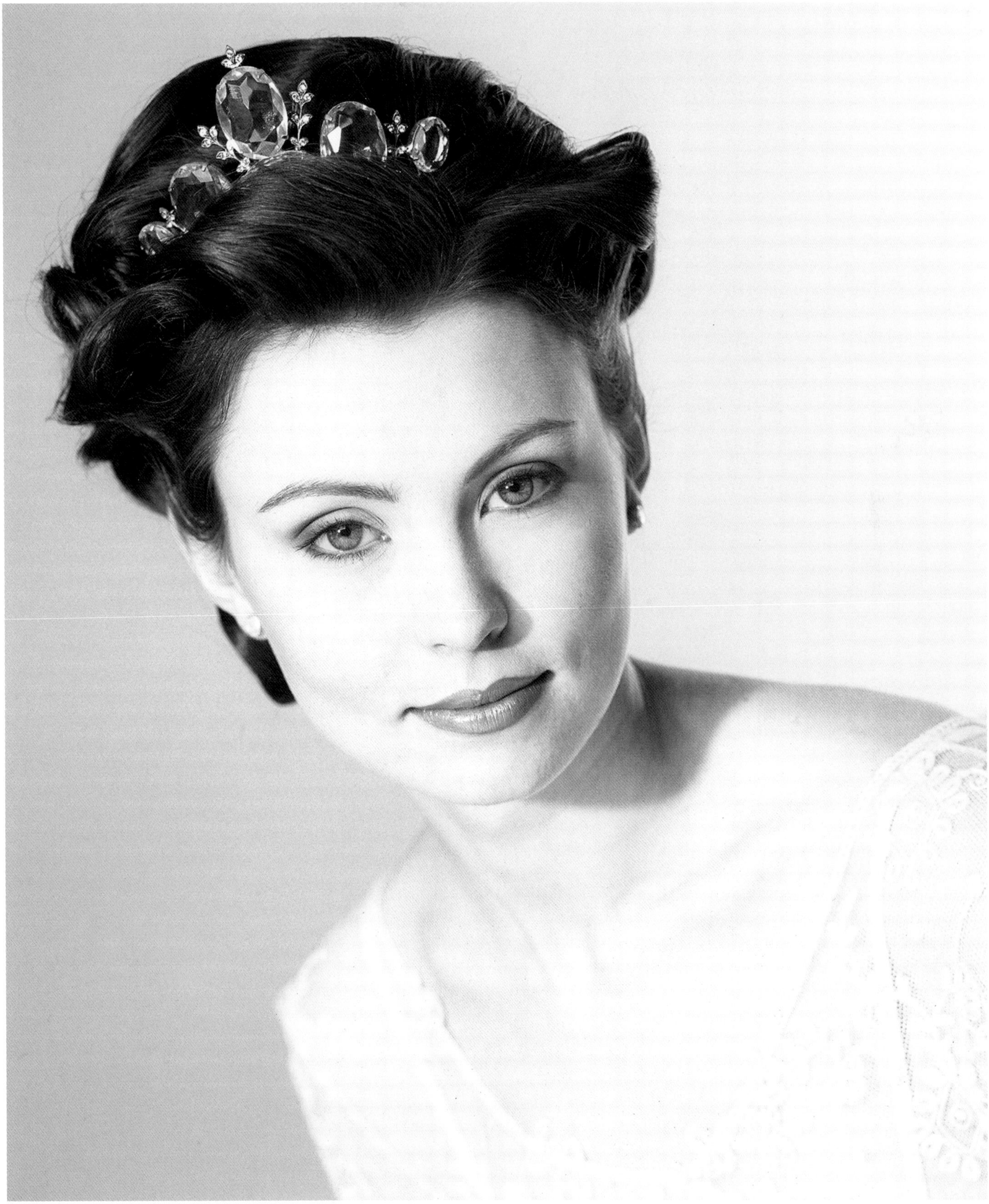

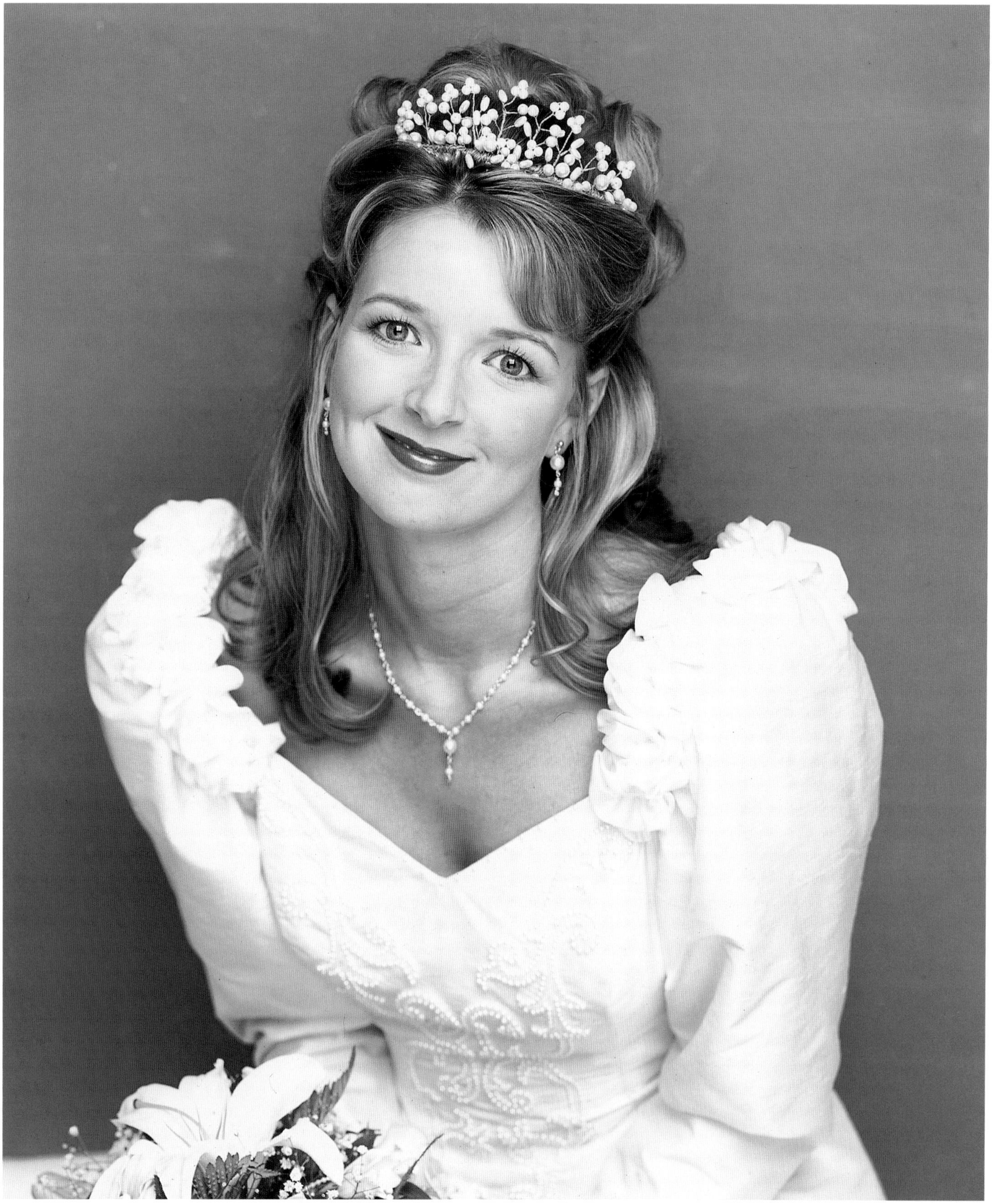

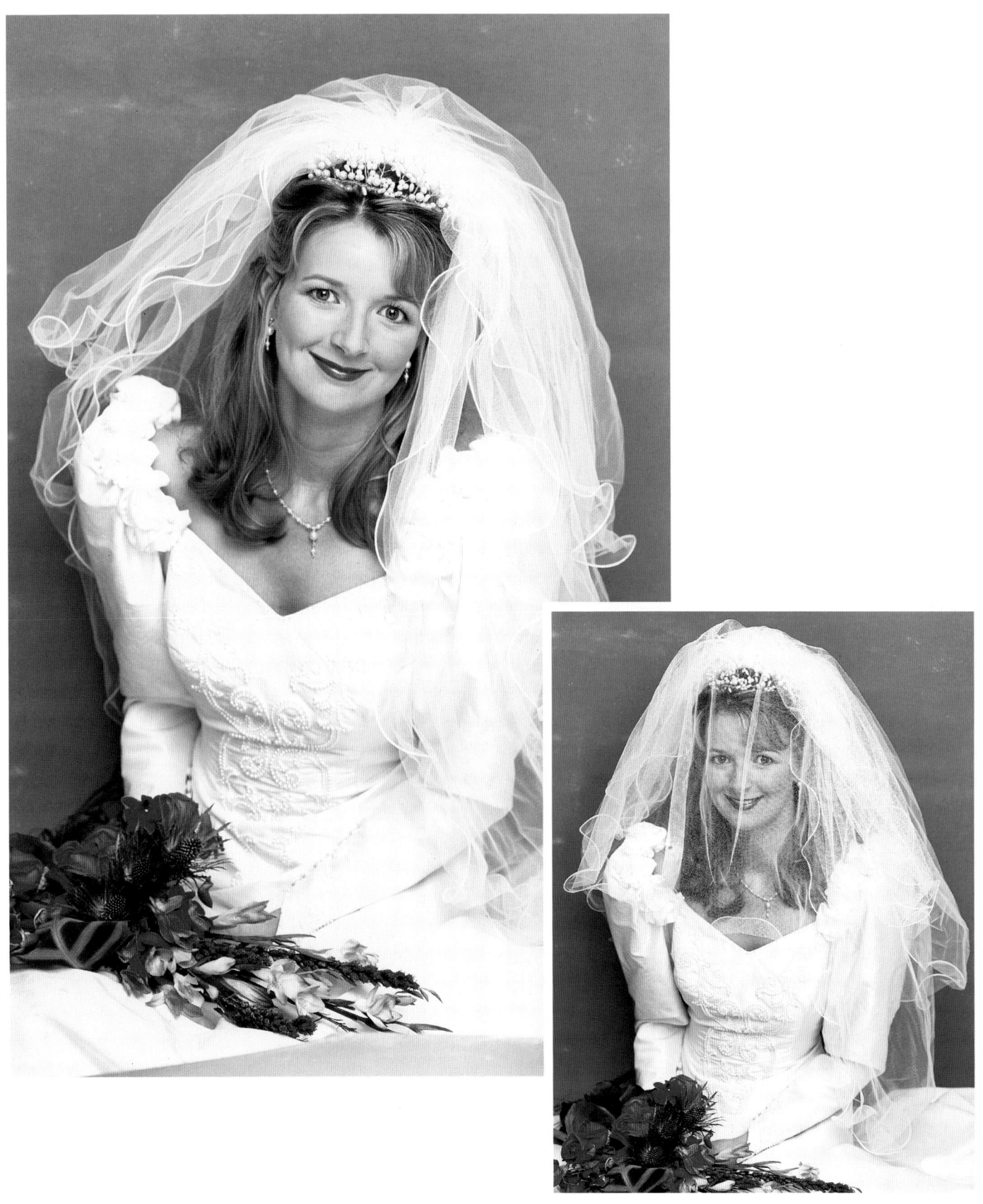

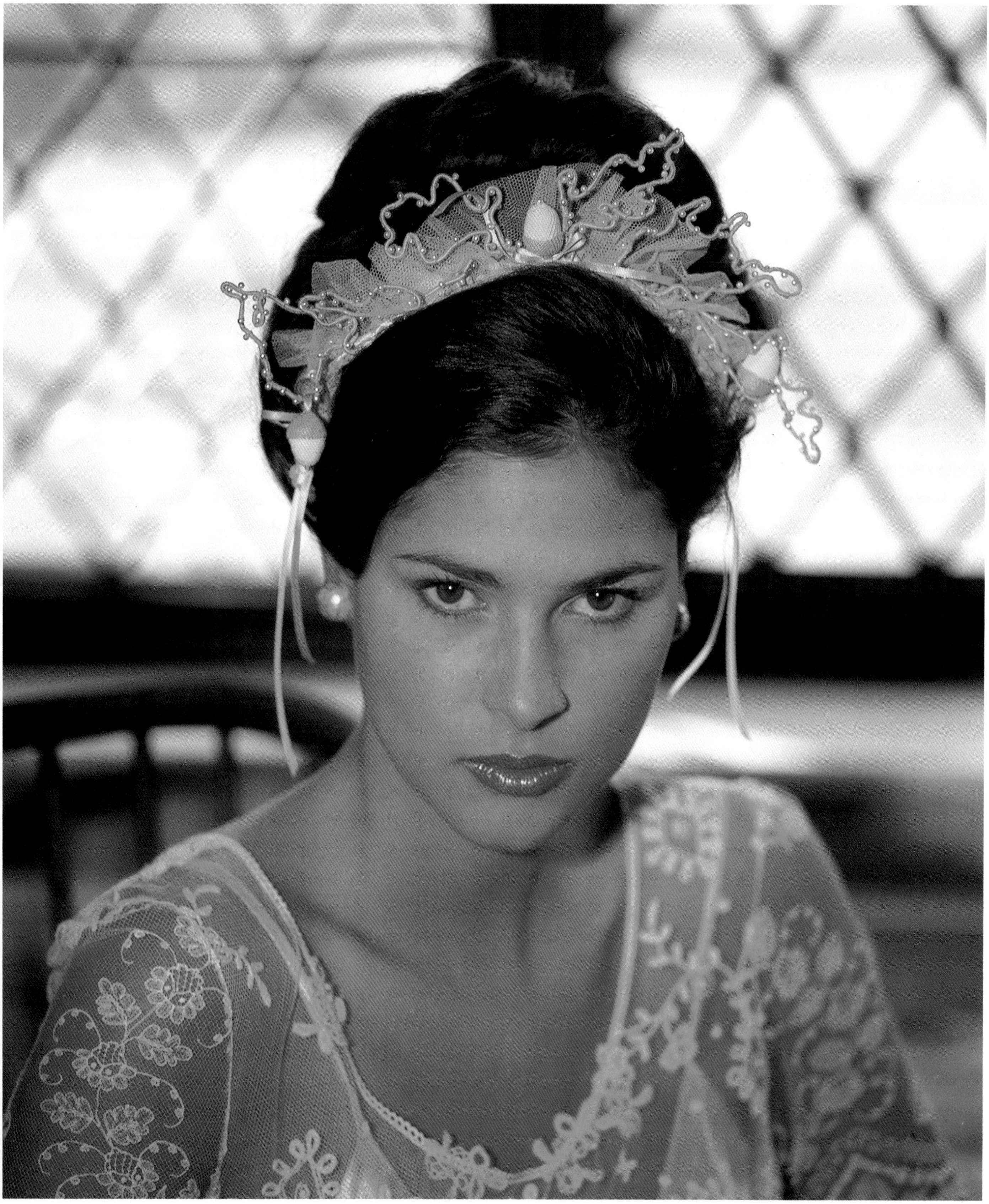

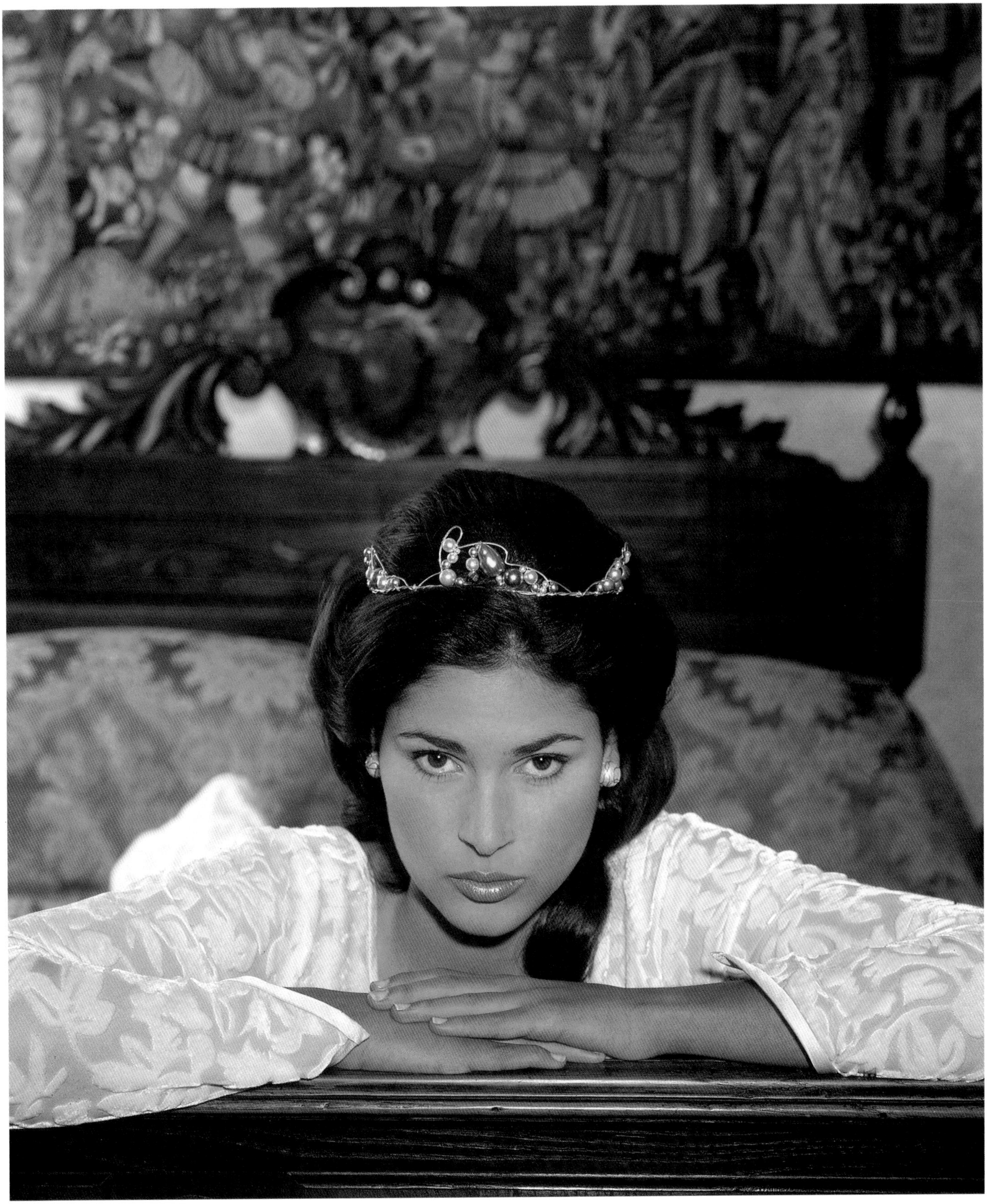

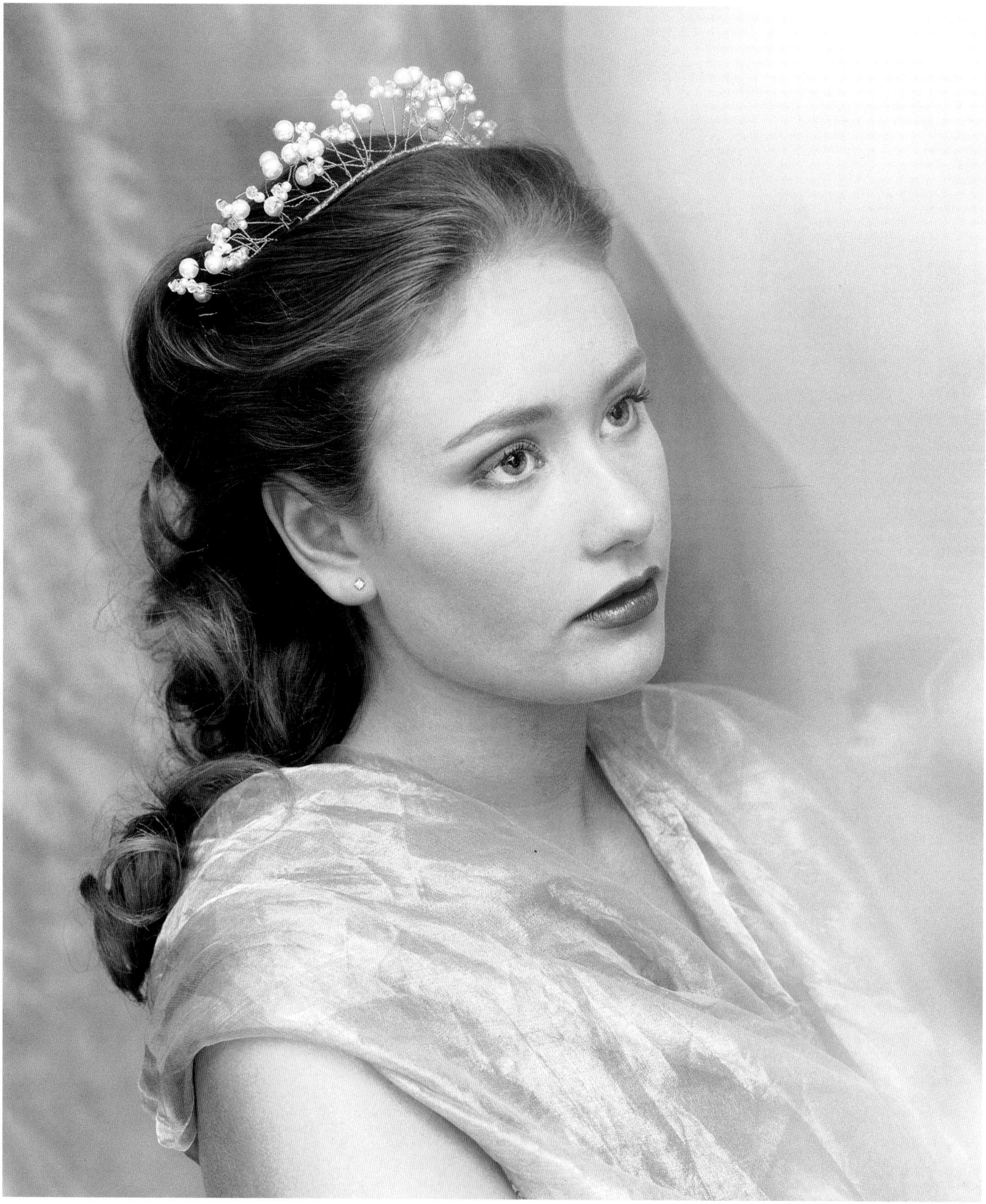

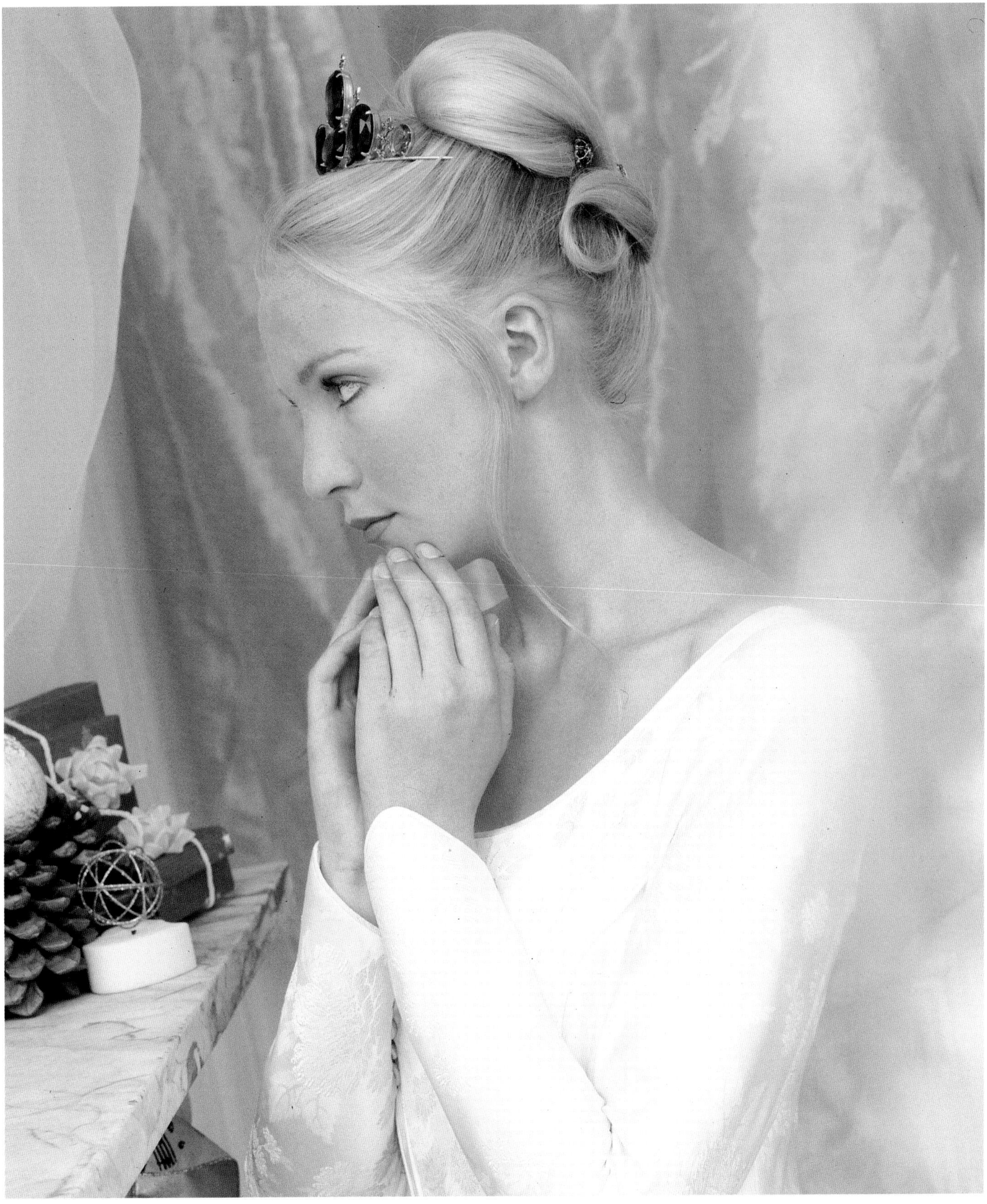

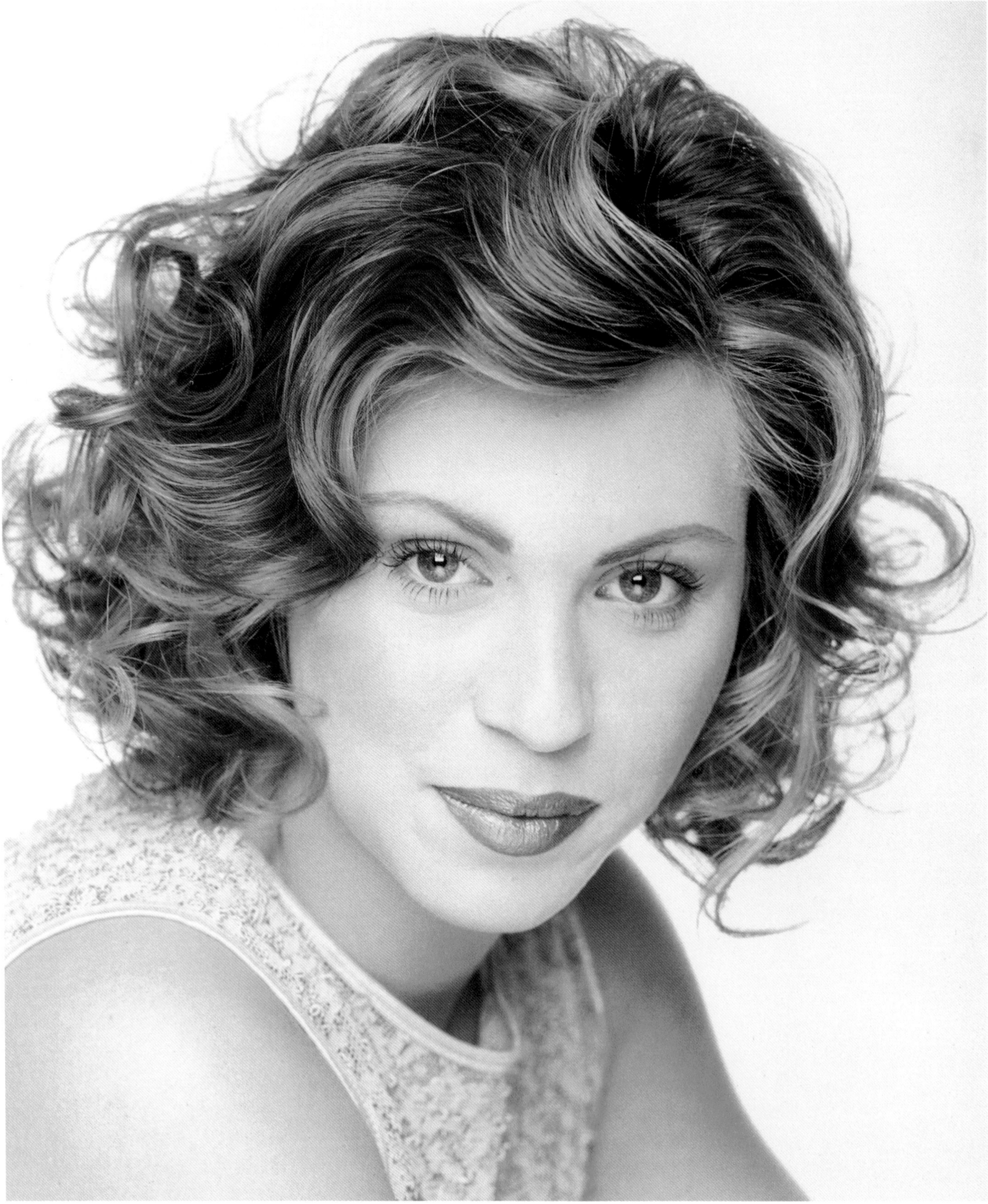

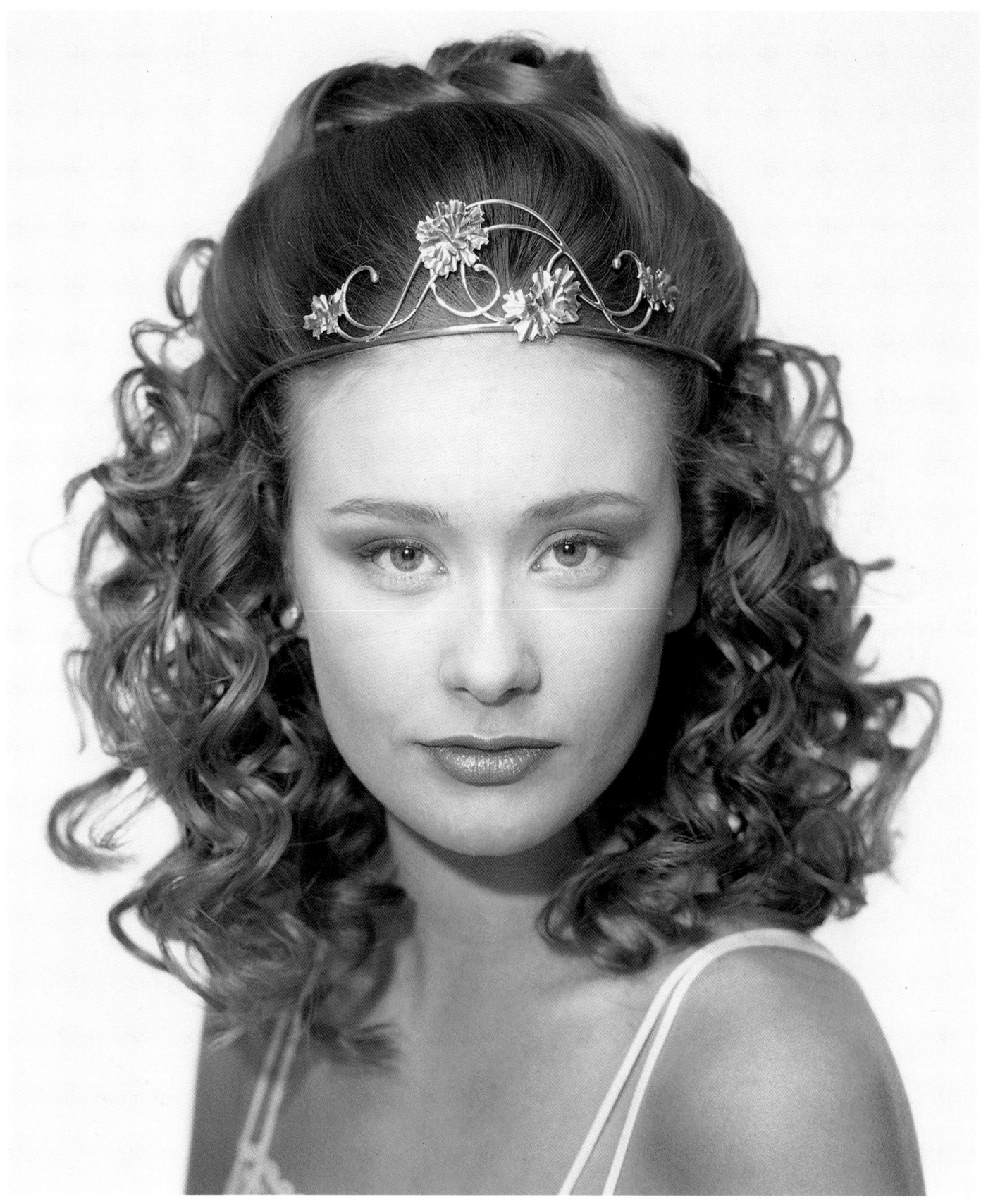

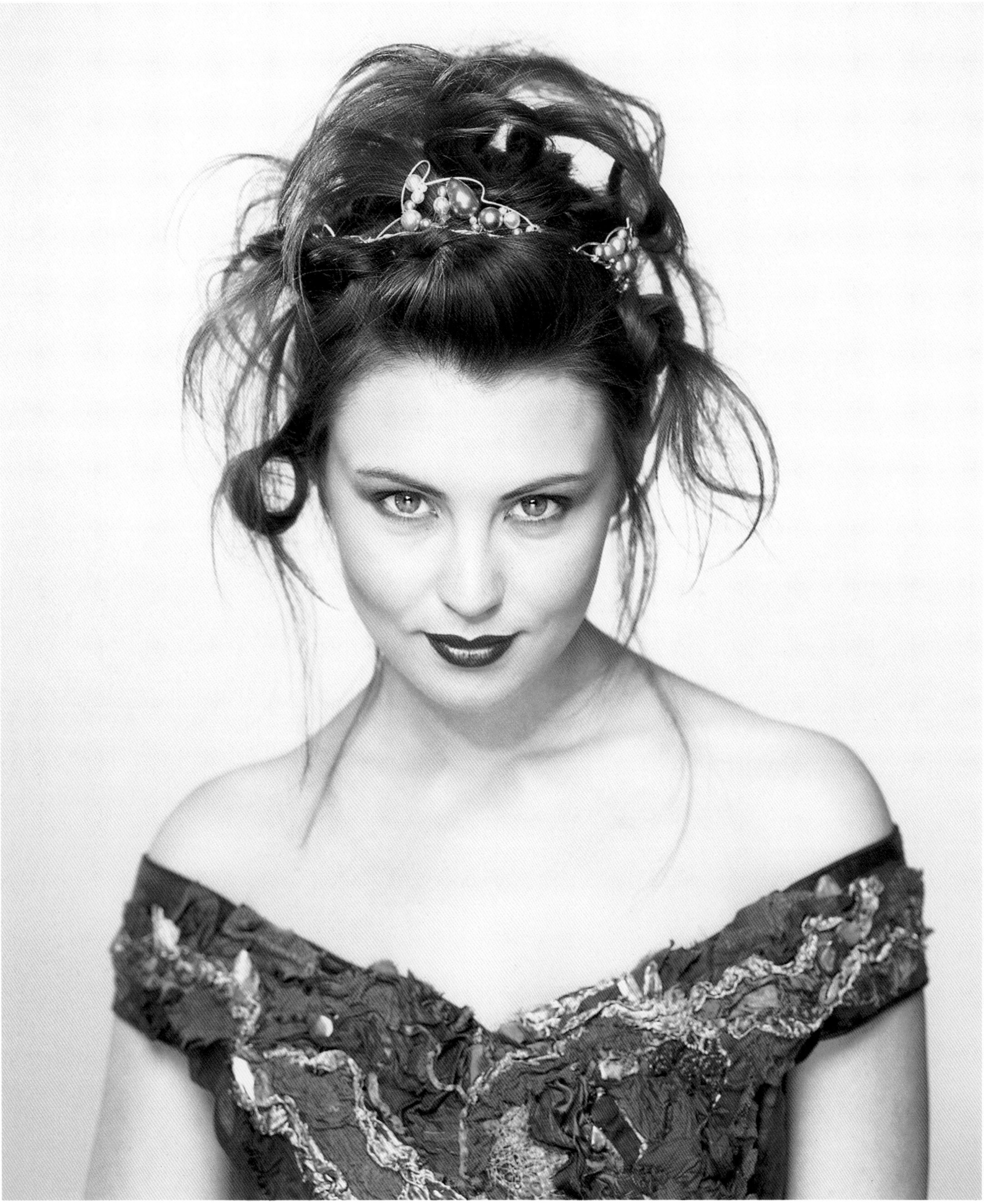

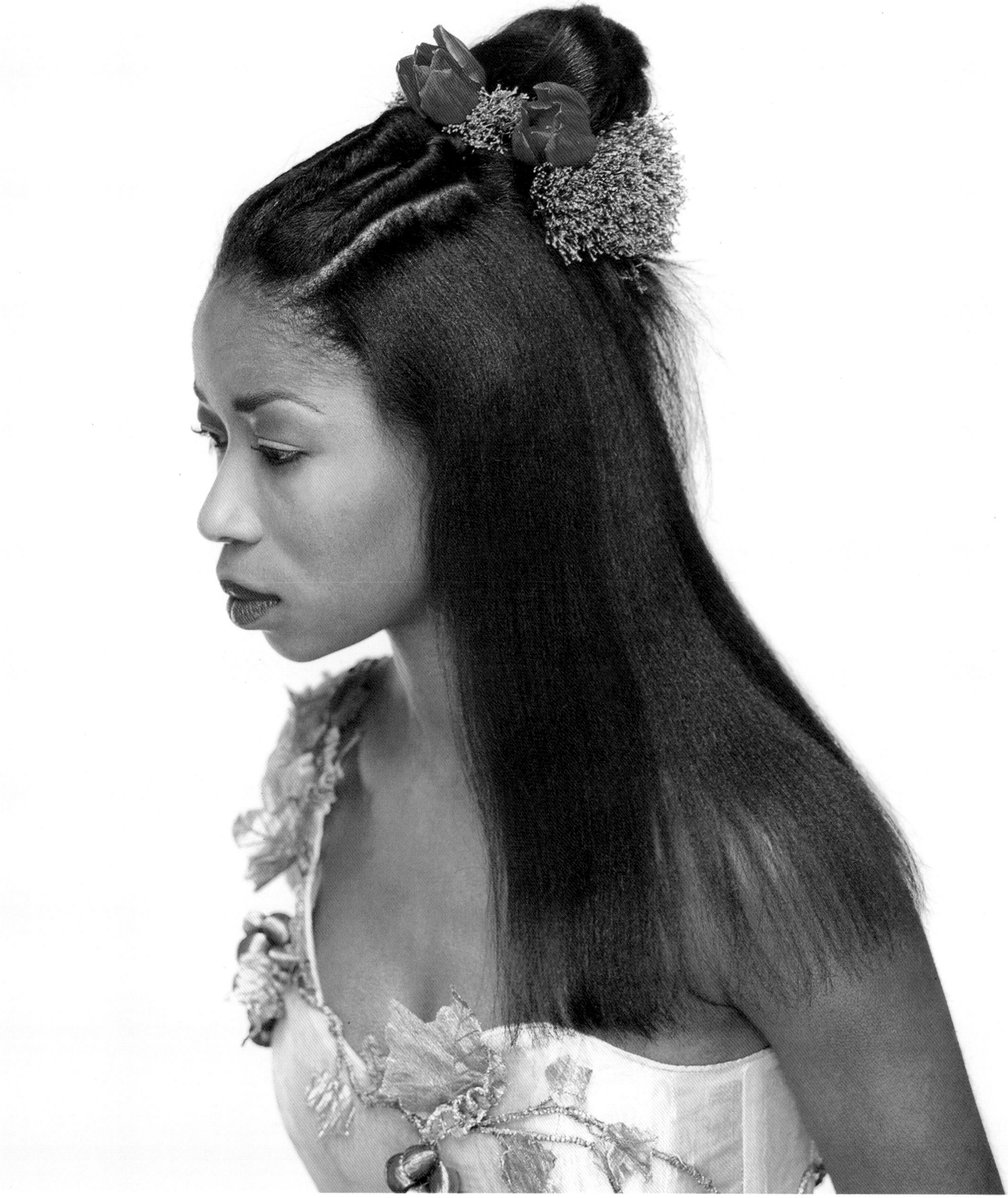

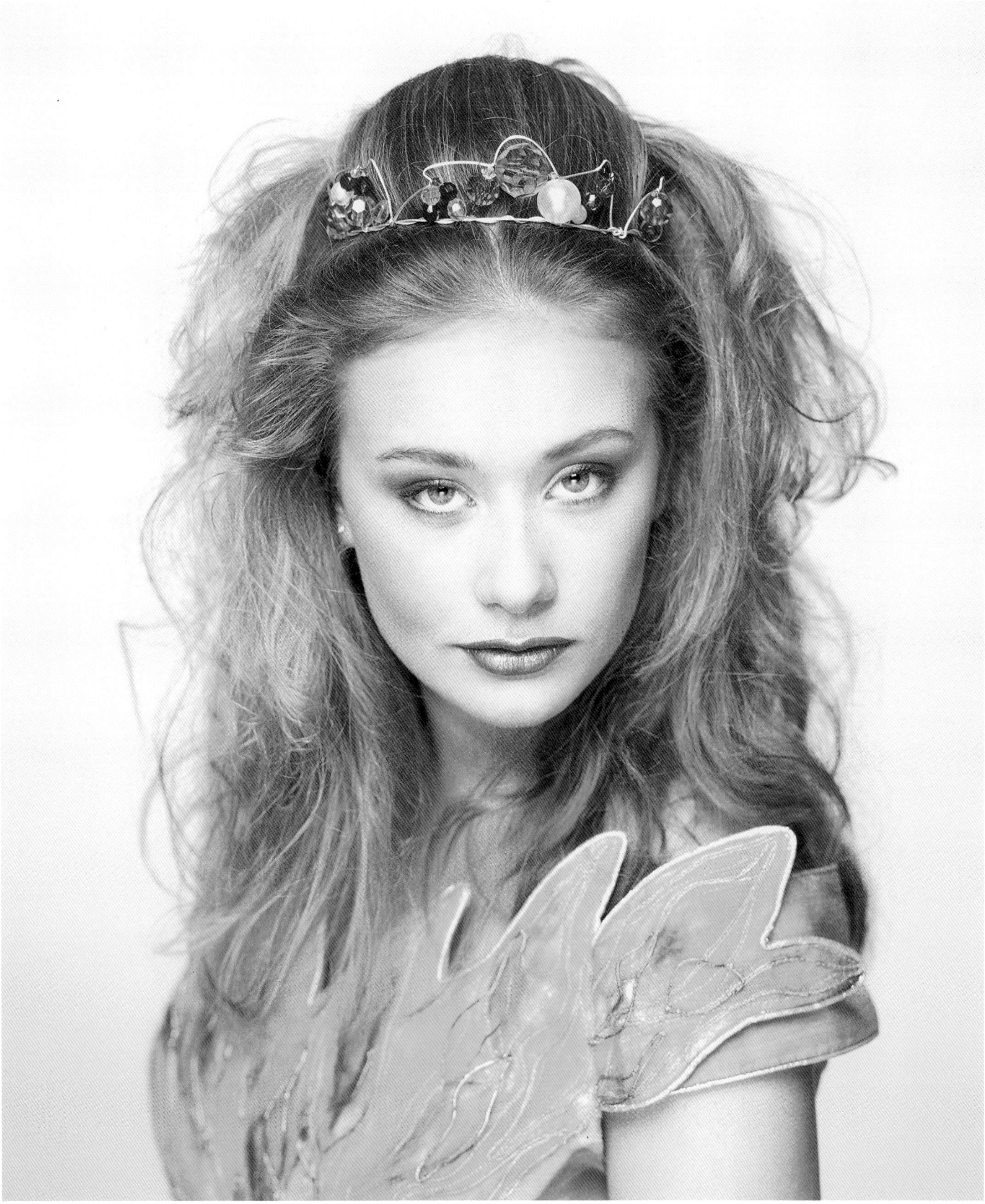

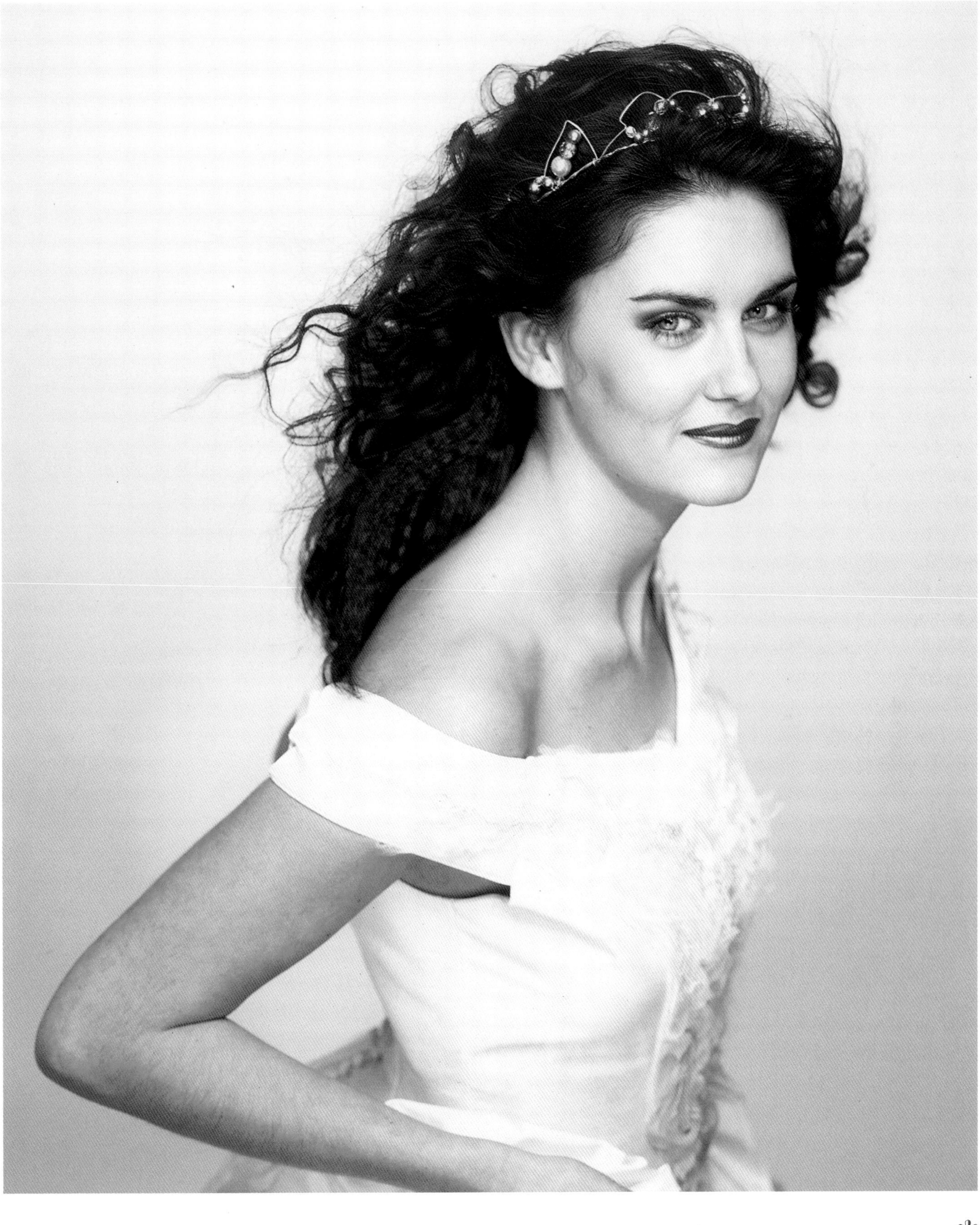

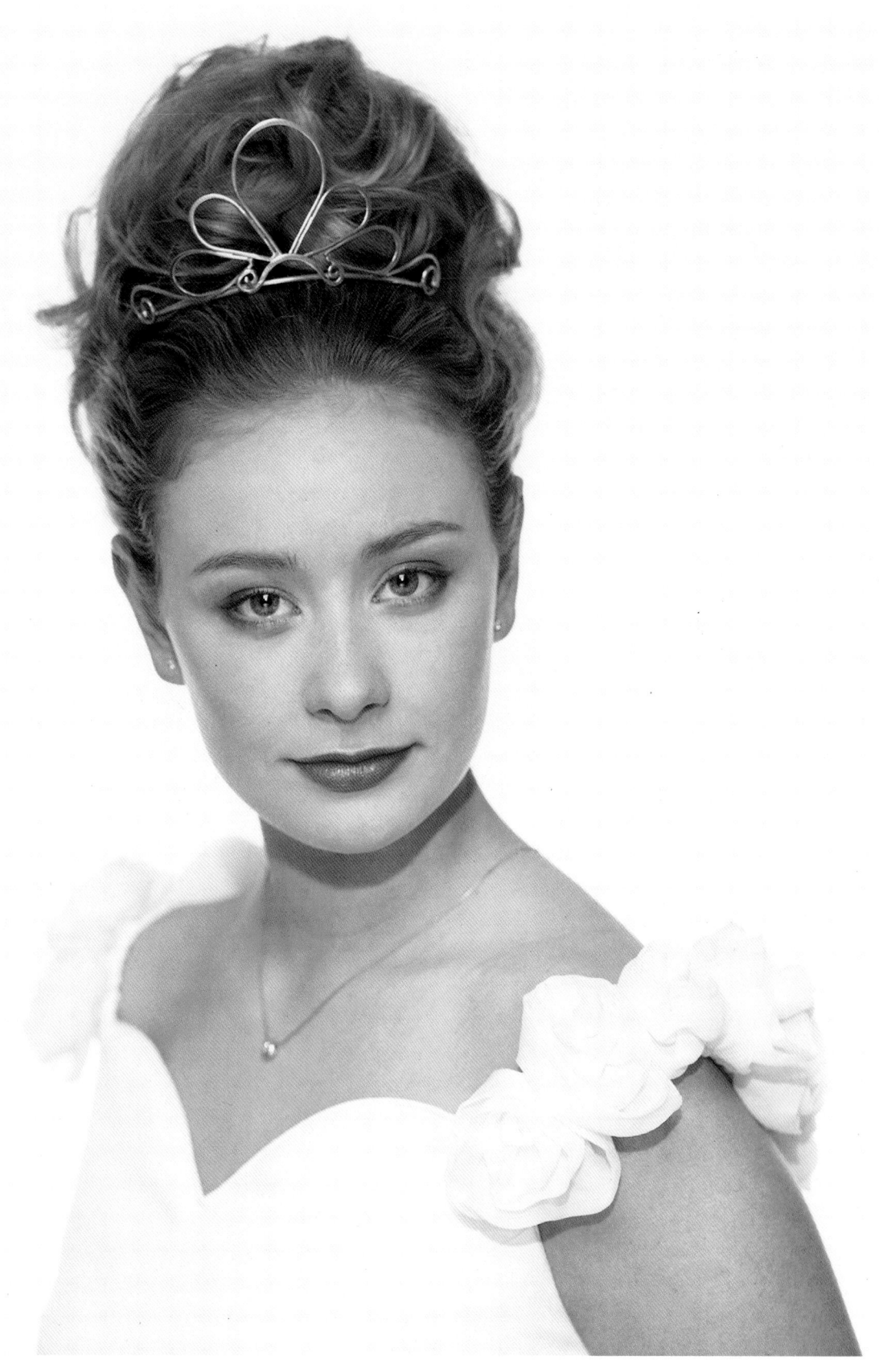

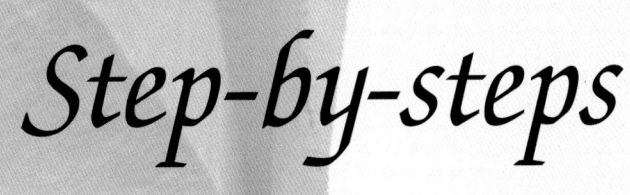

Step-by-steps

14 easy-to-follow techniques

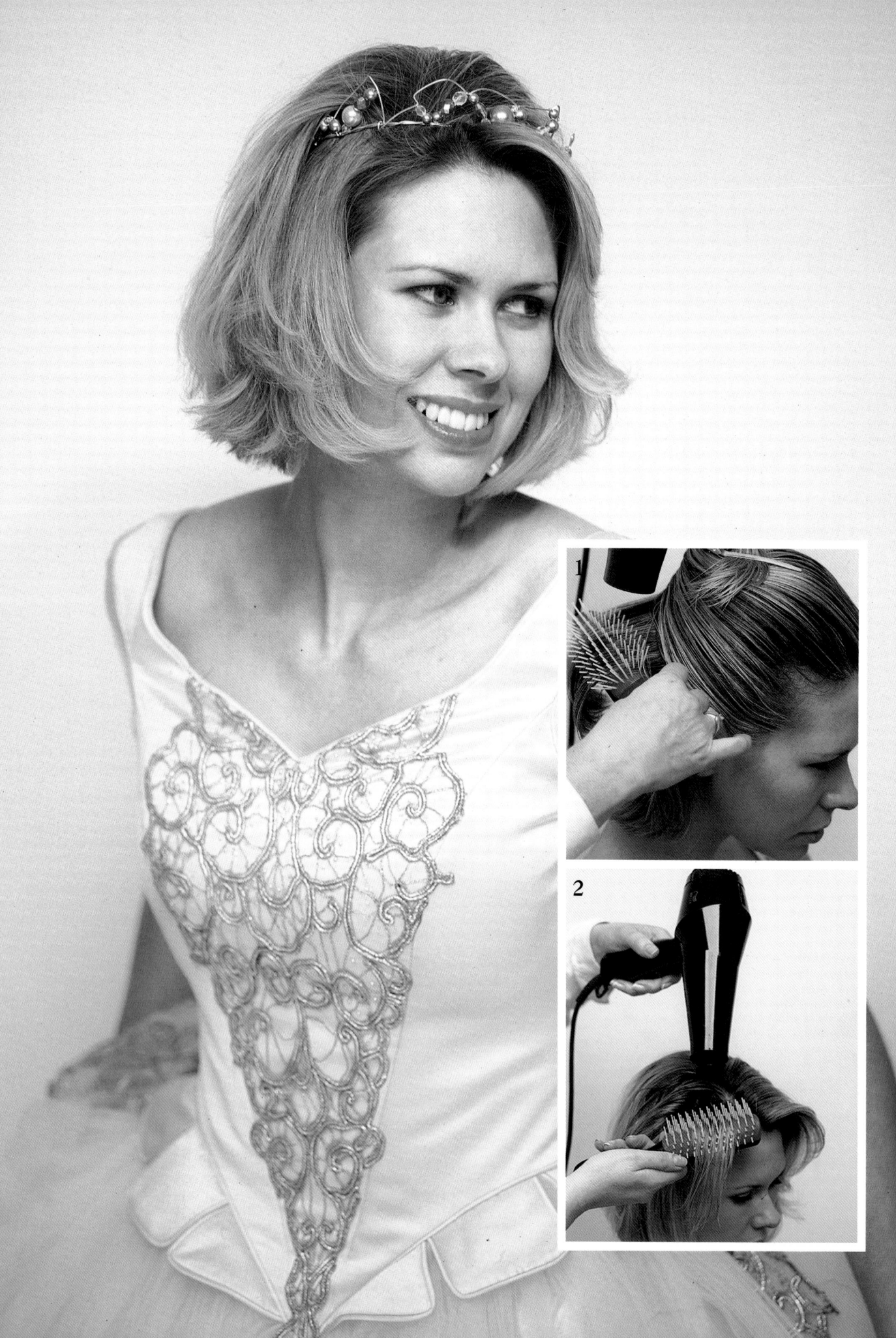

IRIS

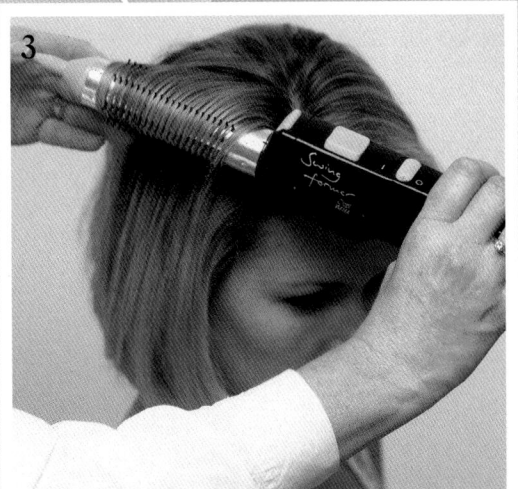

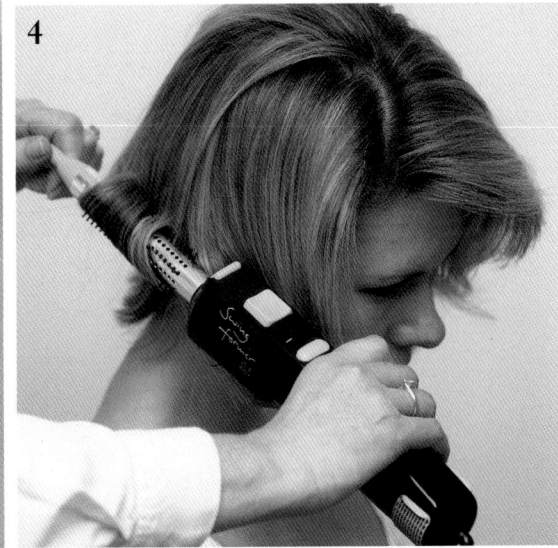

1 Section off top hair and clip out of the way. Blow-dry, lifting hair at root level to achieve volume.

———— ✳ ————

2 Unclip top hair and blow-dry in same manner.

———— ✳ ————

3 Use a hot air styler with a large barrel brush to build body and create smoothness.

———— ✳ ————

4 Flick out ends of hair using a hot air styler with a small barrel brush. Backcomb hair lightly at roots before fixing tiara.

TIP

Point the barrel of the hairdryer so that the warm air flows down the hair shaft. This flattens the cuticle of the hair and helps give a greater shine.

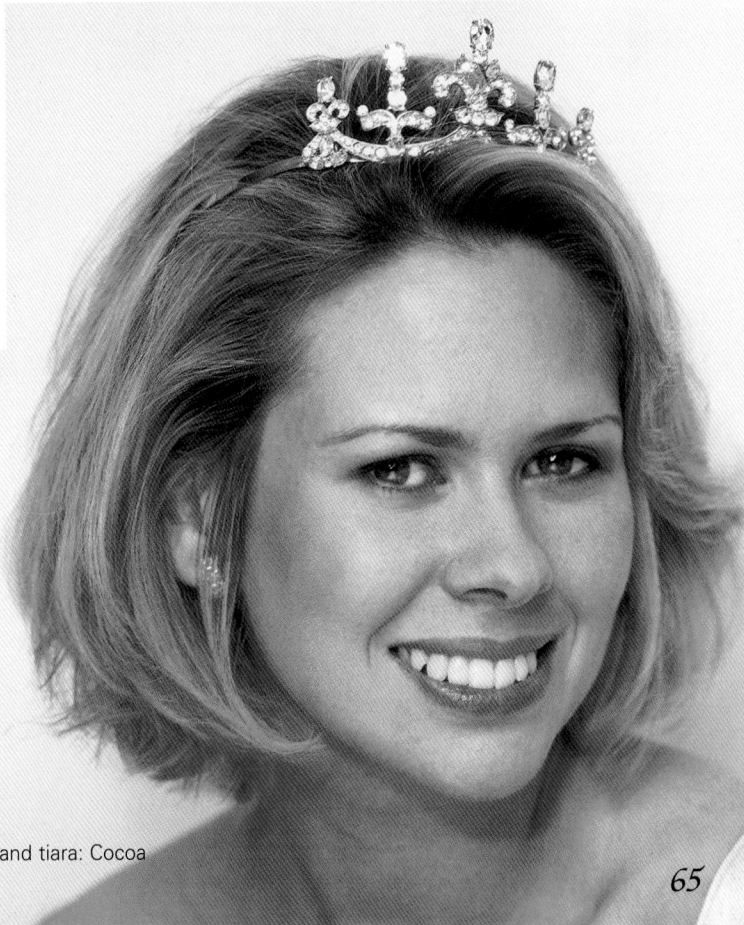

Dress and tiara: Cocoa

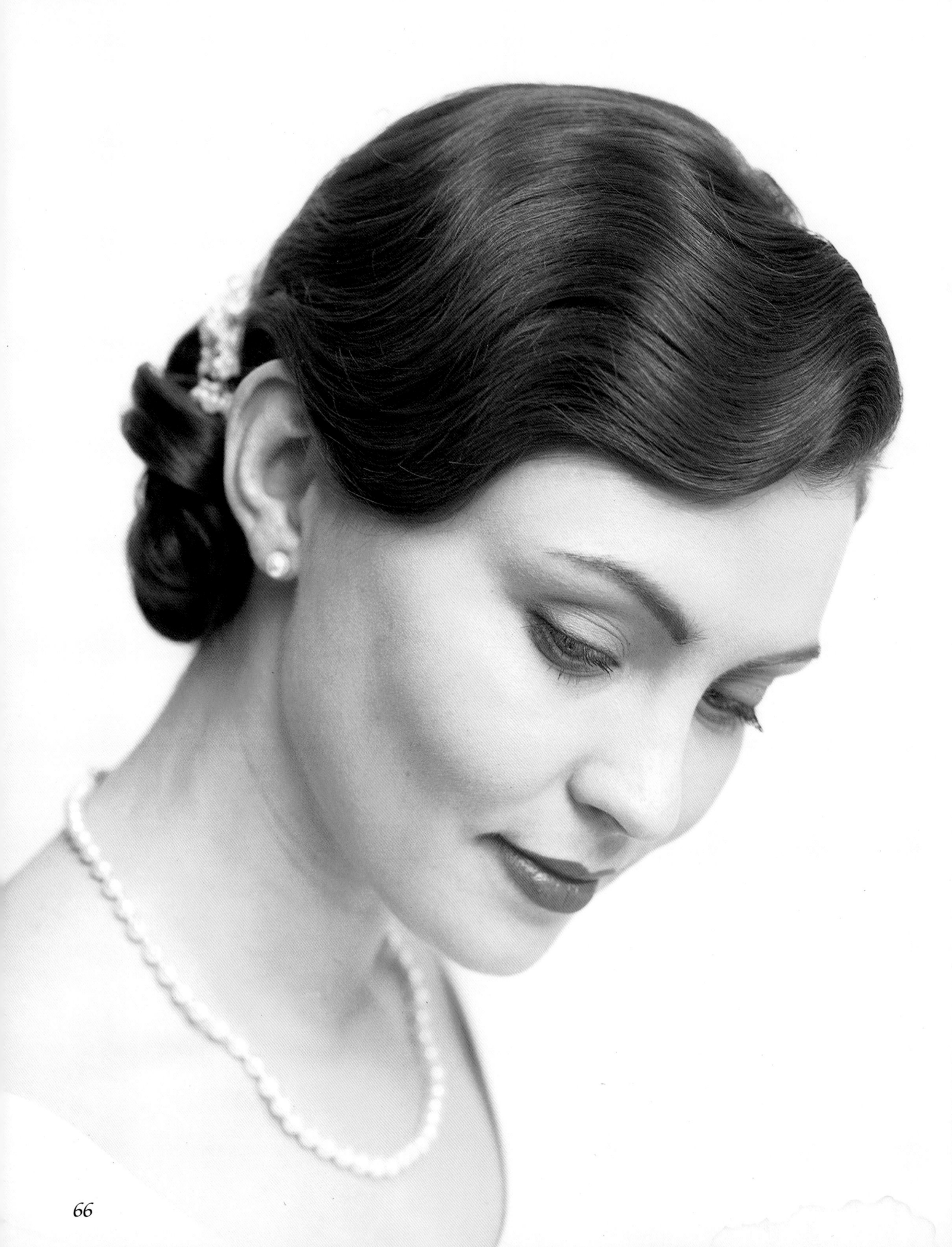

BLOSSOM

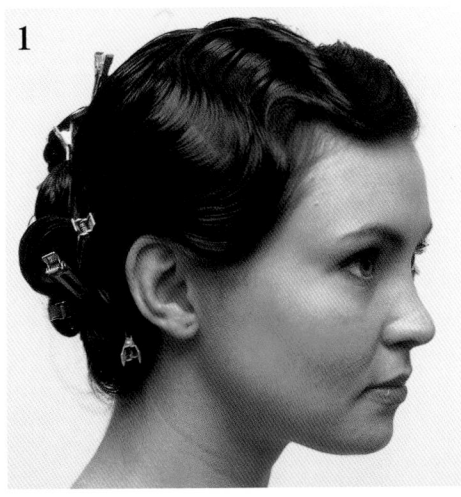

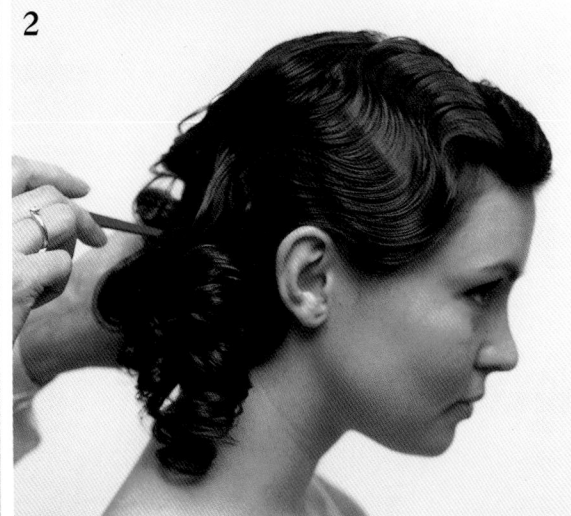

1 Mist hair thoroughly with styling spray. From a side parting, fingerwave front hair and spiral barrel curl back hair. Heat set under a dryer and allow to cool completely.

———— ✳ ————

2 Release barrel curls and allow to fall.

———— ✳ ————

3 Use a bristle brush to gently smooth hair, allowing it to form into gentle waves.

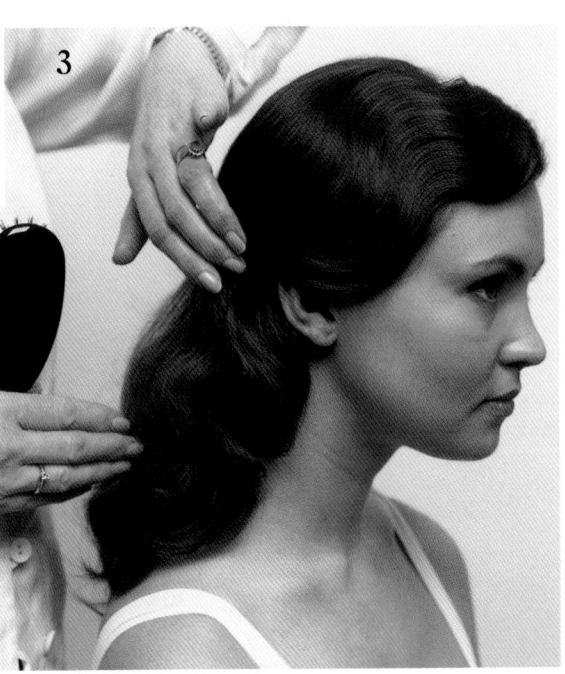

TIP

A bristle brush helps eliminate static and is great for hair that tends to be flyaway.

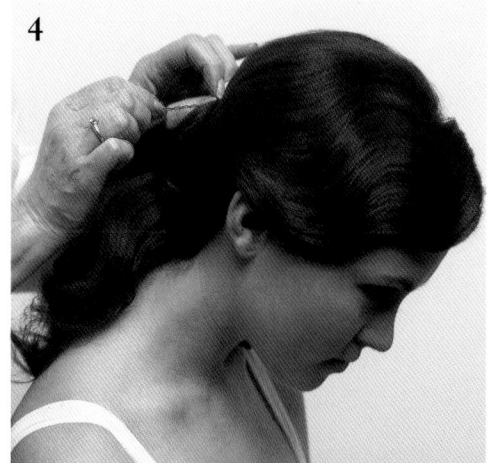

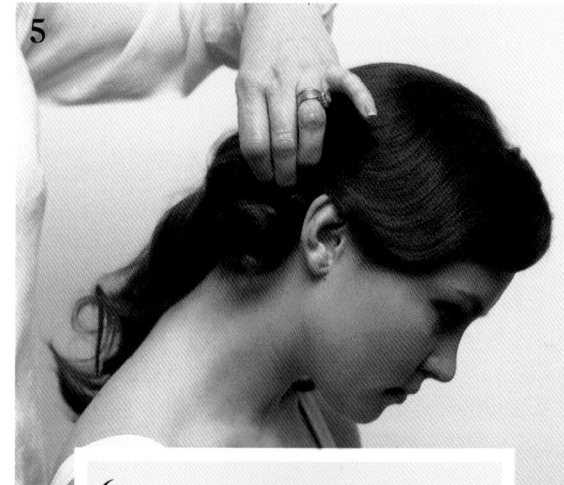

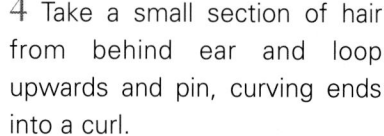

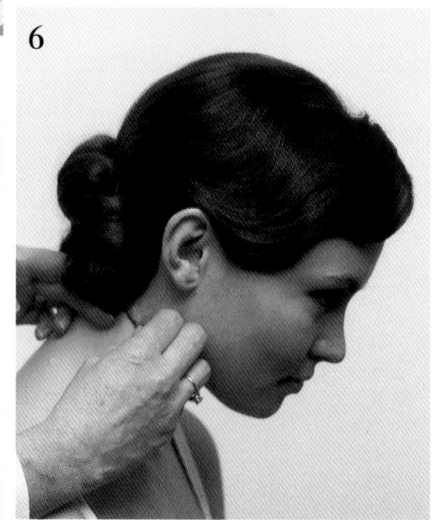

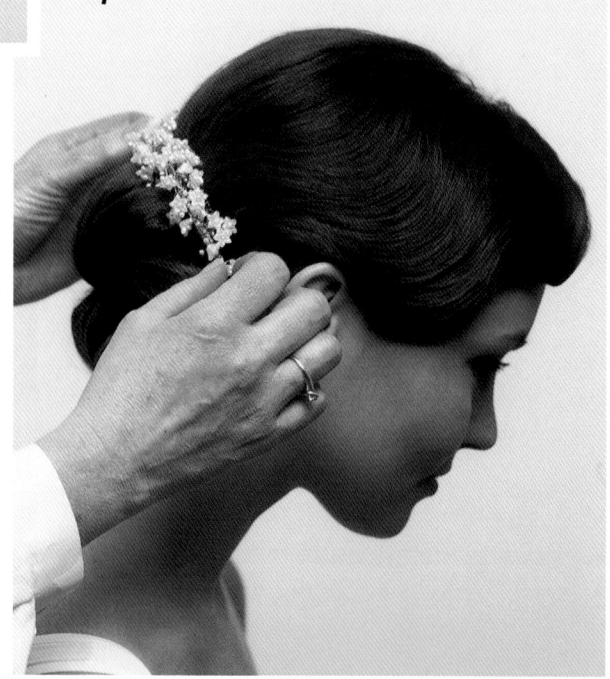

4 Take a small section of hair from behind ear and loop upwards and pin, curving ends into a curl.

———— ✳ ————

5 Take another small section of hair and twist over first curl, allowing ends to hang temporarily free.

———— ✳ ————

6 Secure end of curl at nape of neck using a grip. Dress remaining lengths of hair in same way.

———— ✳ ————

7 Position then grip head-dress in place.

Opposite Head-dress: Classics Bridal Hire Collection

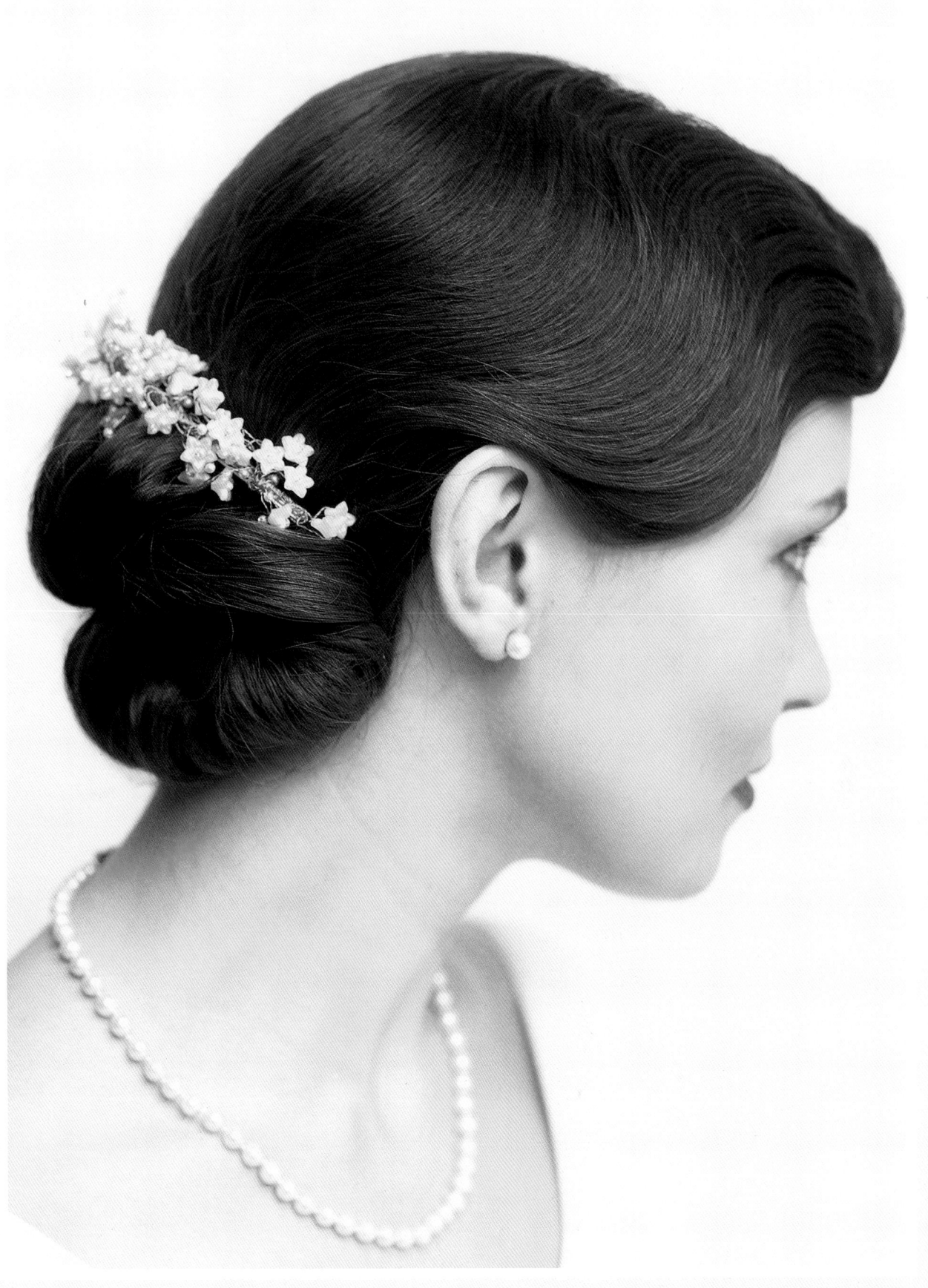

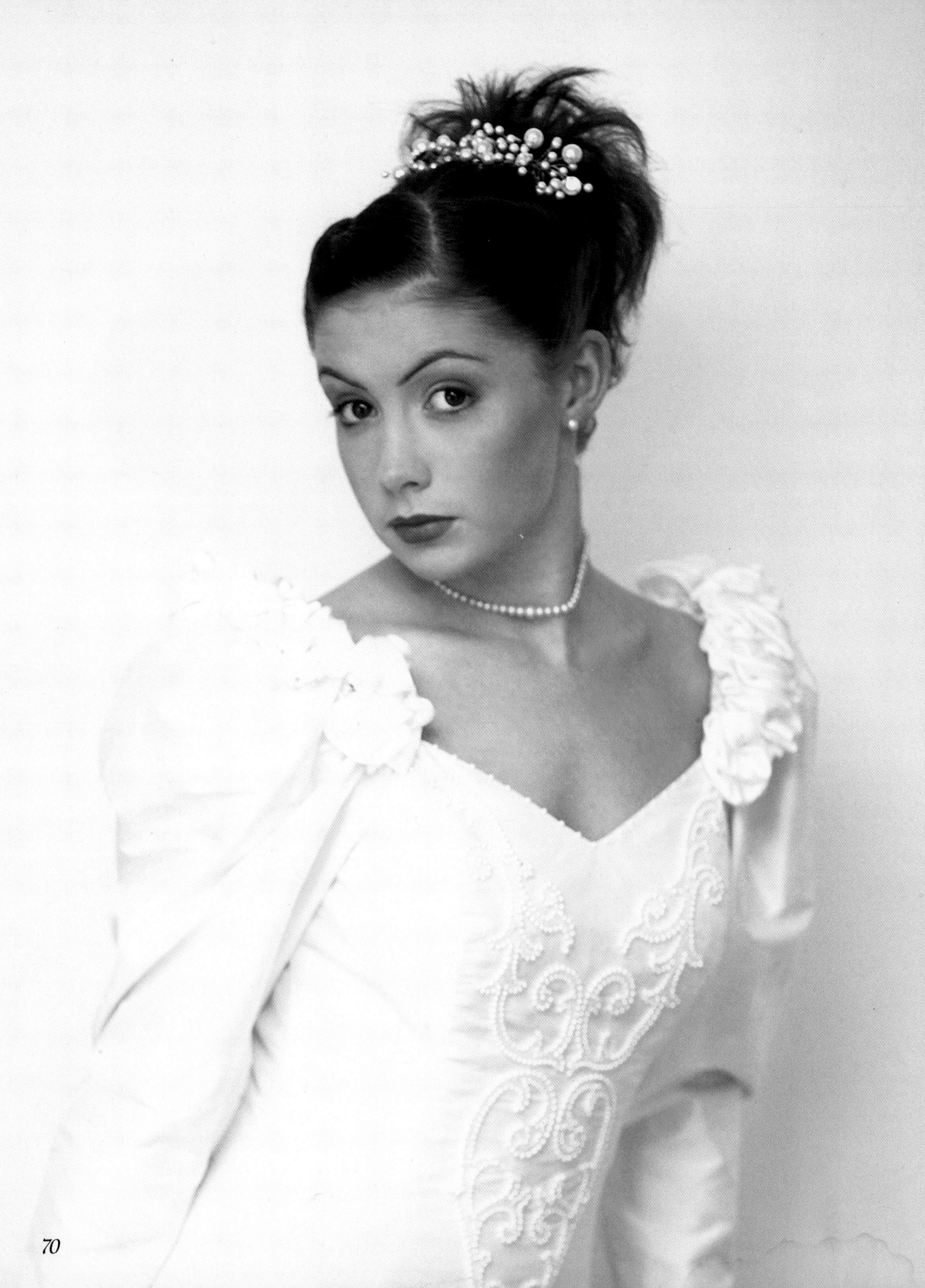

*L*AVENDER

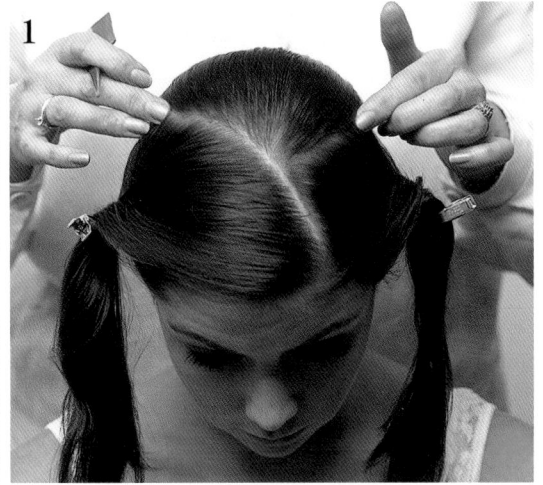

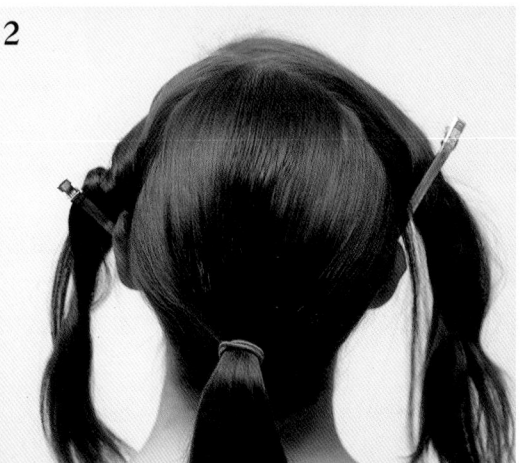

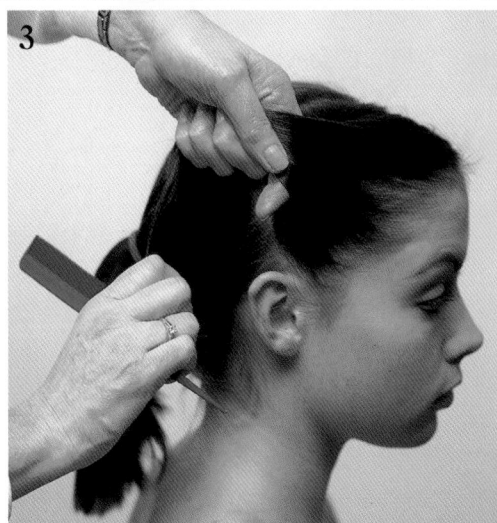

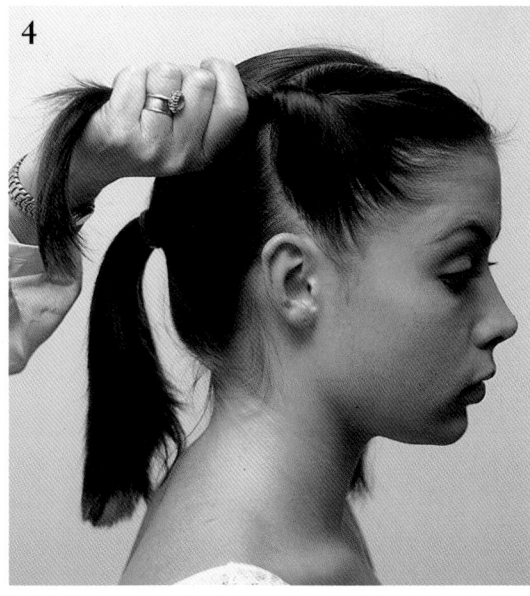

1 Section off front hair from a diagonal parting and secure with section clips. For the time being, secure back hair into a low ponytail and leave until you are ready to work on this section.

———— ✳ ————

2 Shows back view of sectioned hair.

———— ✳ ————

3 Take one side section of hair and mist with styling spray. Comb hair and sweep backwards, placing finger under the point you want the twist to start.

———— ✳ ————

4 Twist this section of hair towards the head, holding tension.

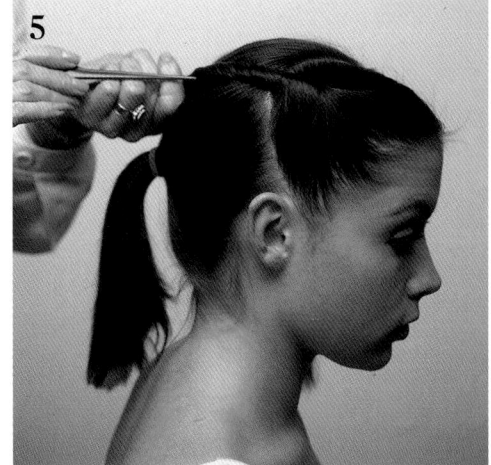

5 Continue twisting, smoothing any stray ends with a tail comb.

———— ✳ ————

6 Secure twist with a hairgrip at back of head.

———— ✳ ————

7 Repeat for other side.

———— ✳ ————

8 Fold ends of twists upwards and grip. Mist with hairspray.

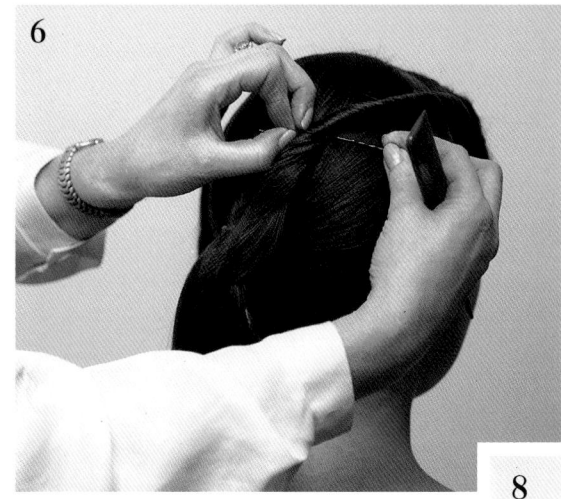

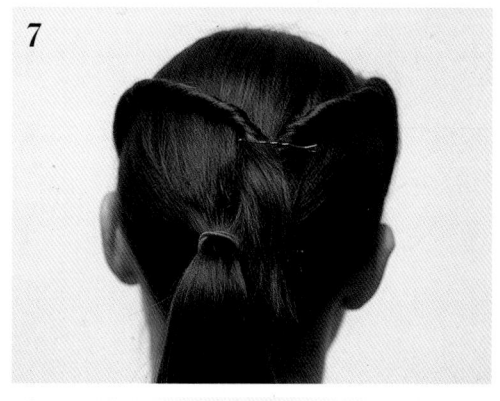

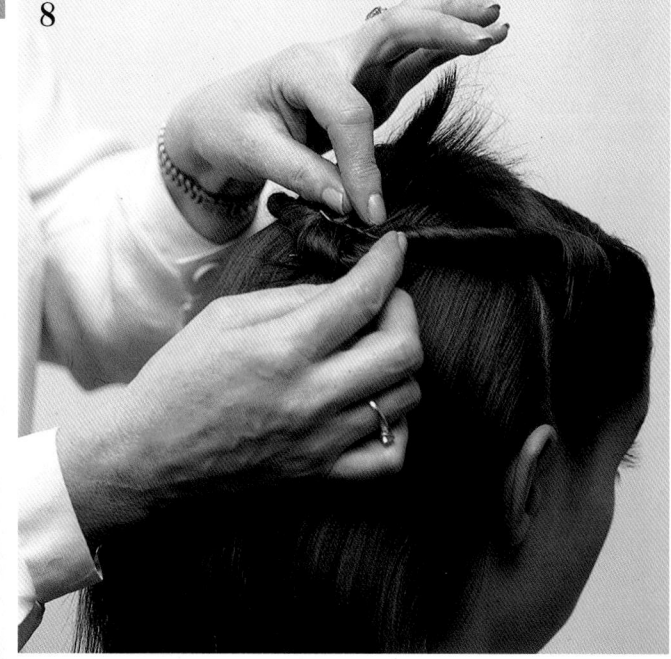

TIP

Use a firm hold hairspray for this style to ensure it stays in place all day.

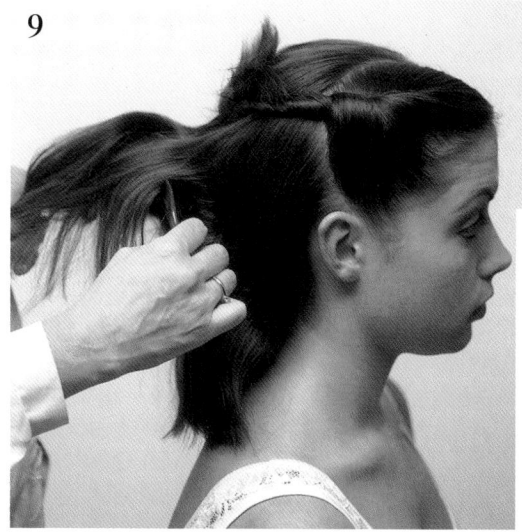

9

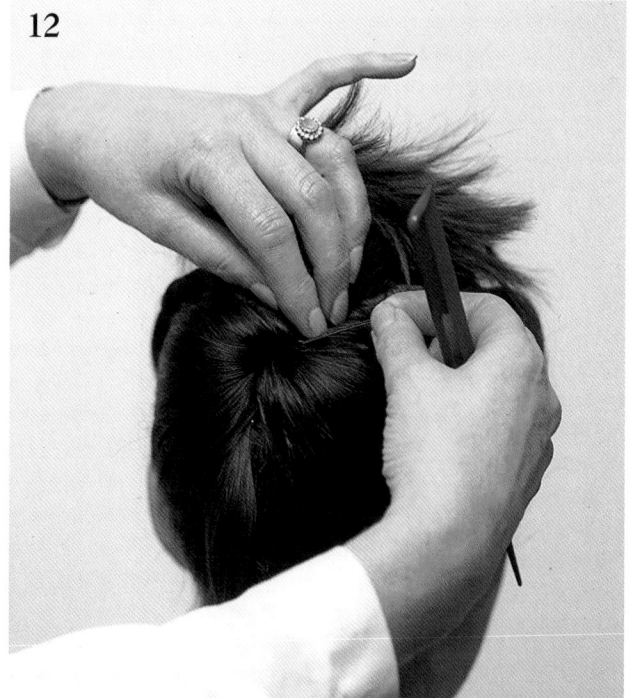

12

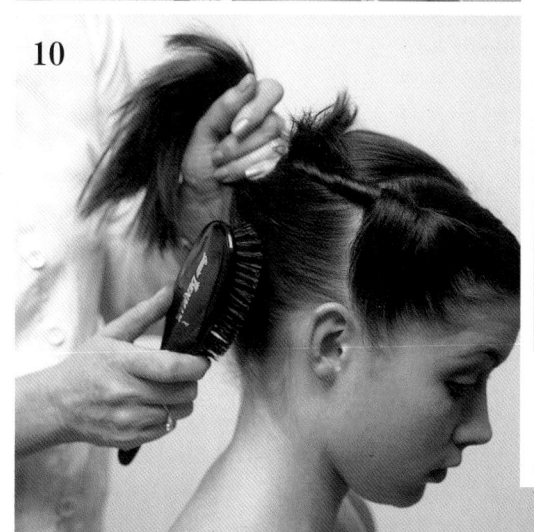

10

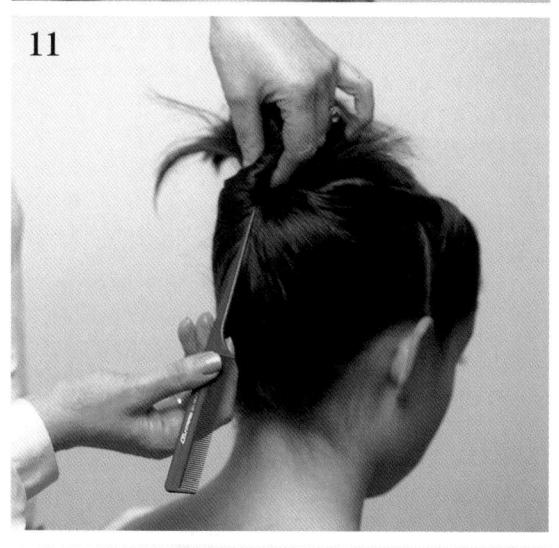

11

9 Release hair from ponytail and lightly backcomb.

———— ✳ ————

10 Use a bristle brush to smooth hair upwards, as if into a high ponytail. Mist with hairspray, making sure all flyaway ends are smoothed into place.

———— ✳ ————

11 Twist hair, allowing ends to fan out.

———— ✳ ————

12 Grip to secure.

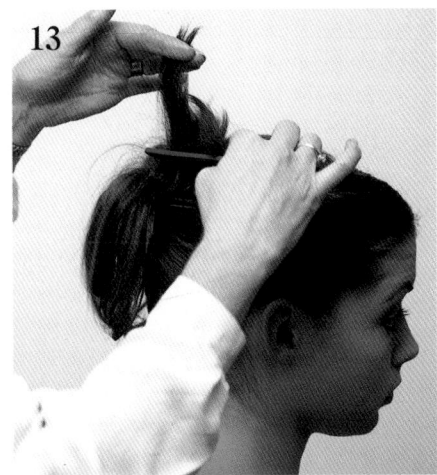

13 Lightly backcomb ends of hair.

———— ✳ ————

14 Mist with hairspray, lifting ends to achieve texture.

———— ✳ ————

15 Take head-dress with a comb attachment. Align teeth of comb centrally on crown of head.

———— ✳ ————

16 Slide comb of head-dress into place.

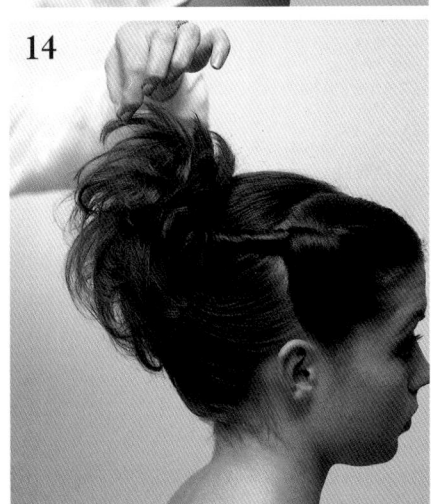

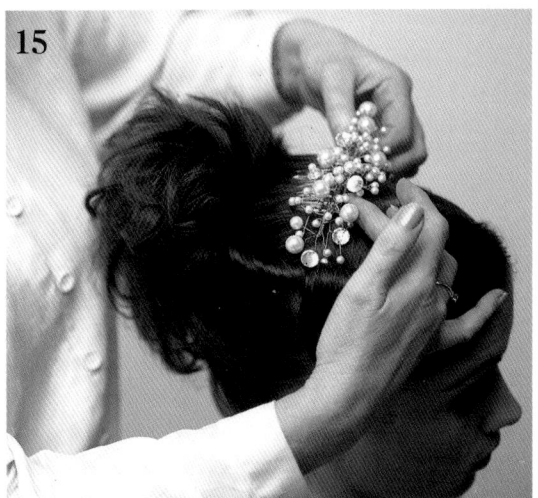

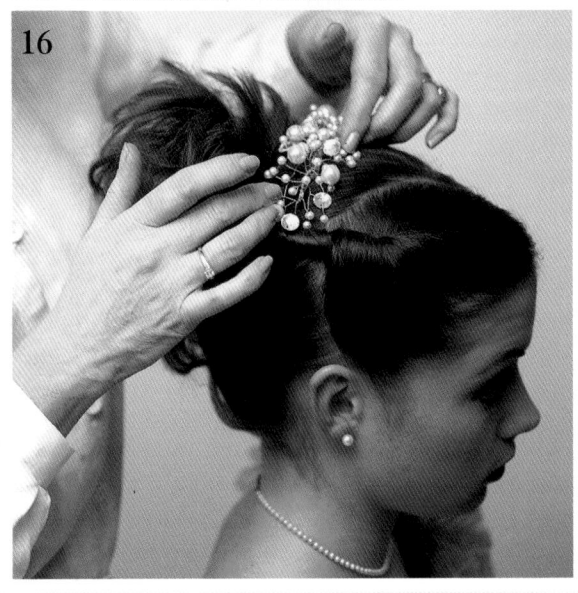

Opposite Dress and head-dress: Classics Bridal Hire Collection

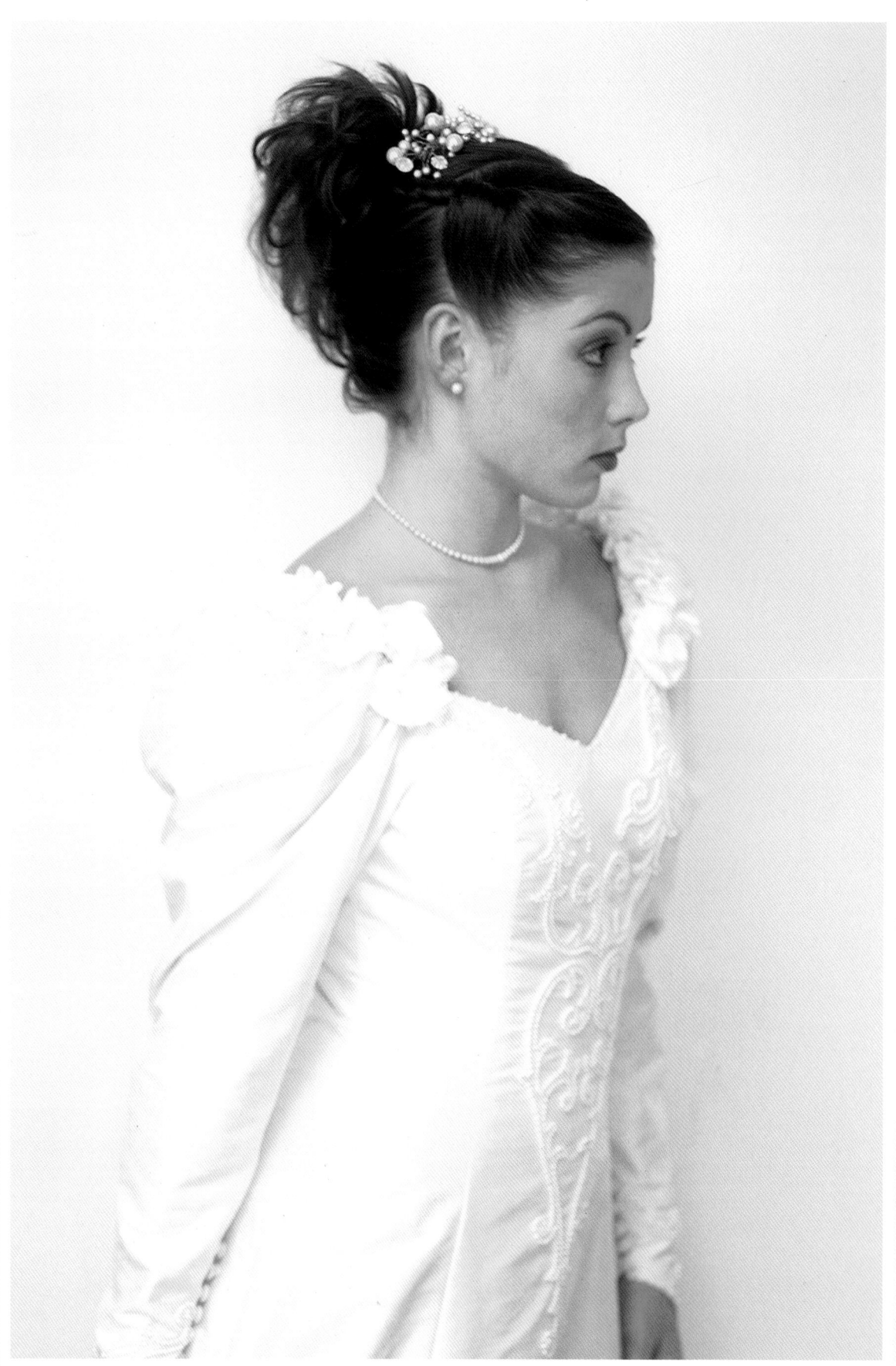

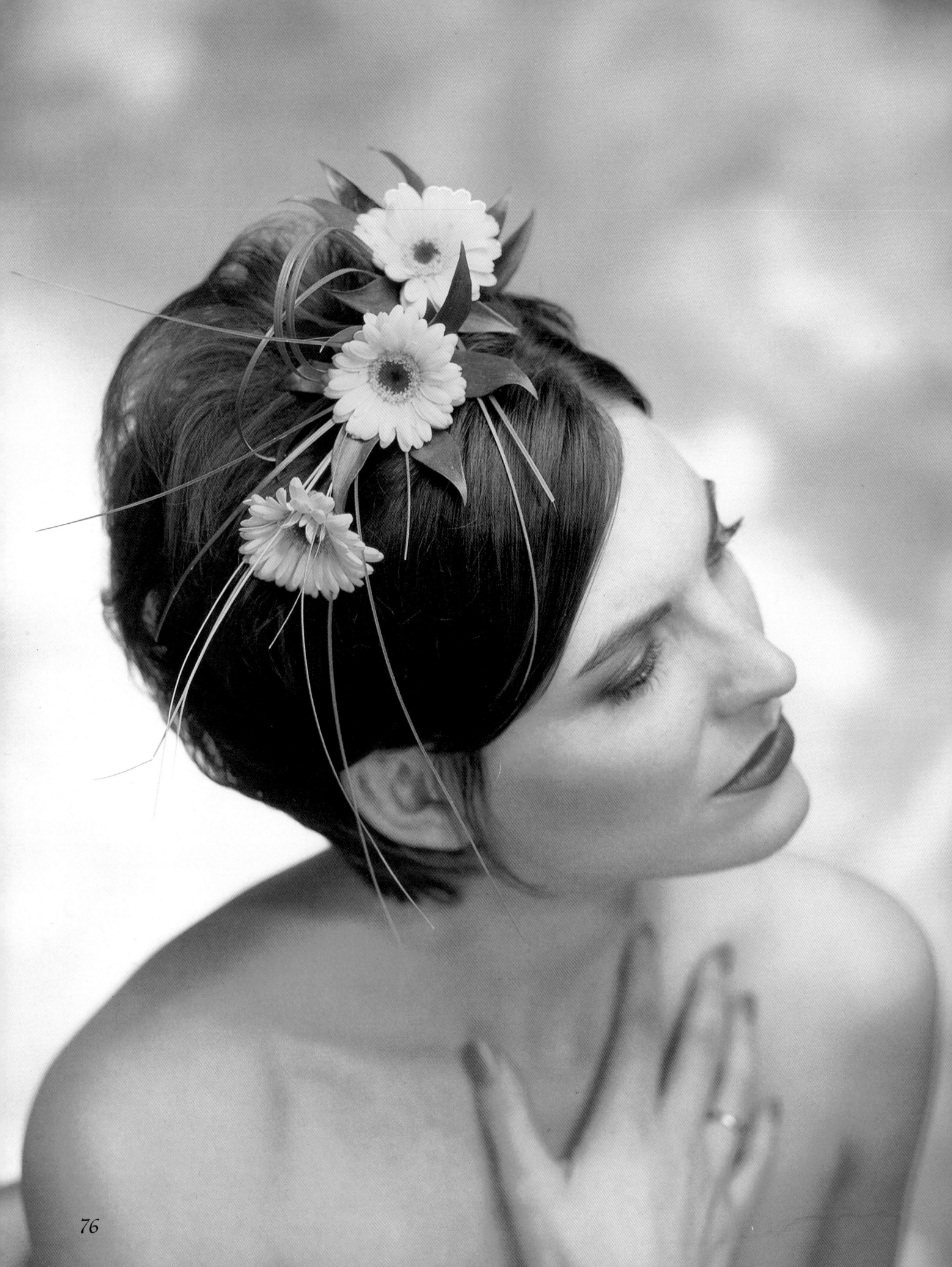

CRYSTAL

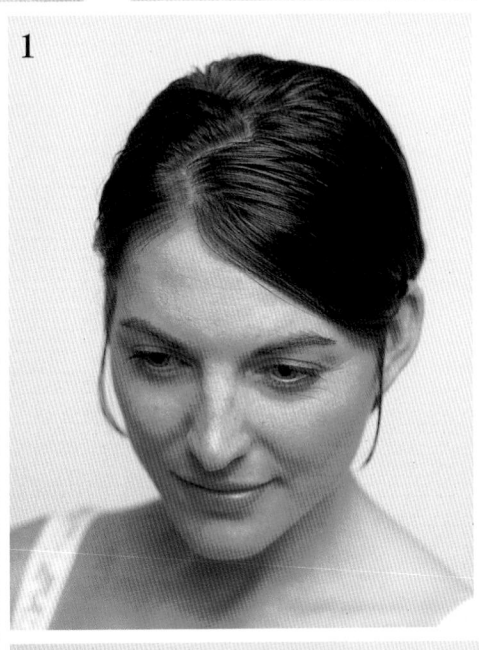

1 Part hair in a zig-zag line, leaving side tendrils free.

———— * ————

2 Blow-dry lower hair, using the minimum amount of styling product, so you maintain the maximum shine on the hair.

———— * ————

3 Use a hot air styler to achieve volume on crown.

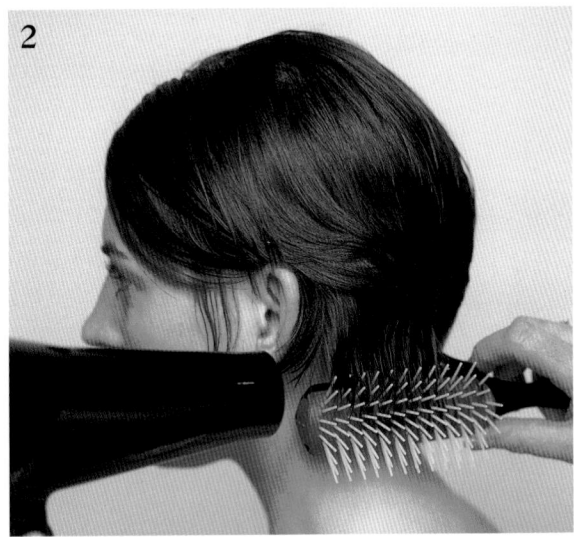

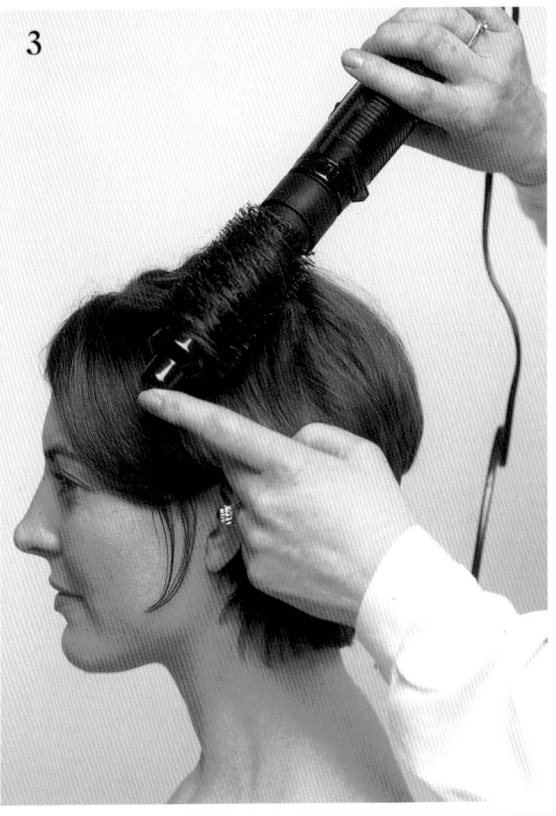

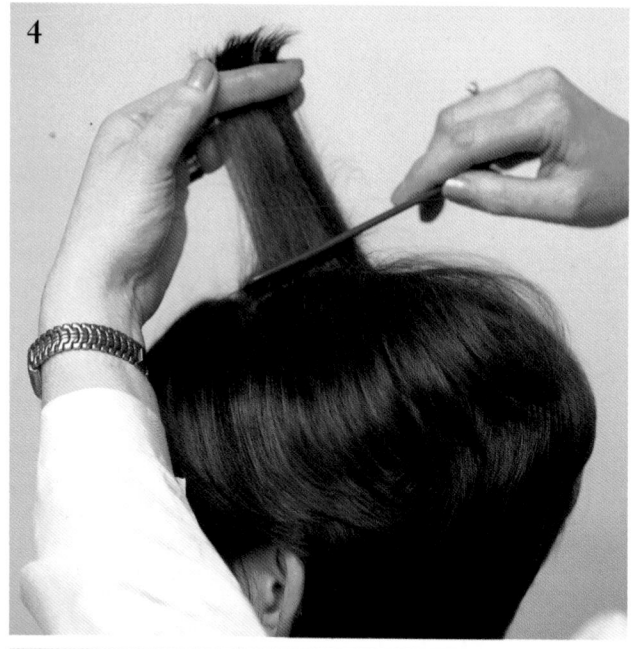

4 Lightly backcomb crown hair at roots to give height and provide a good base for attaching the floral head-dress.

———— ✳ ————

5 Grip head-dress in place.

———— ✳ ————

6 Apply a little gel to side tendrils and curve onto face.

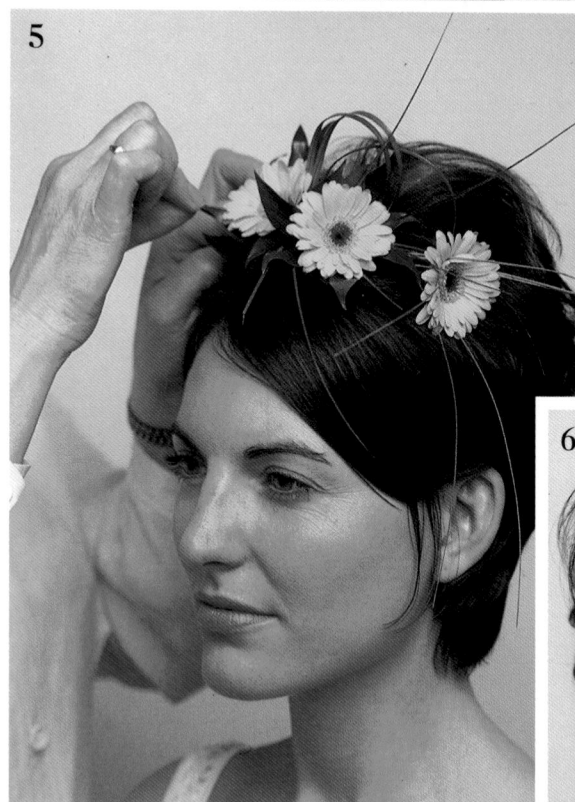

✳ ———————— ✳

𝒯IP

By combining the use of a hot air styler and backcombing hair at the roots you will ensure that the floral head-dress stays in place.

✳ ———————— ✳

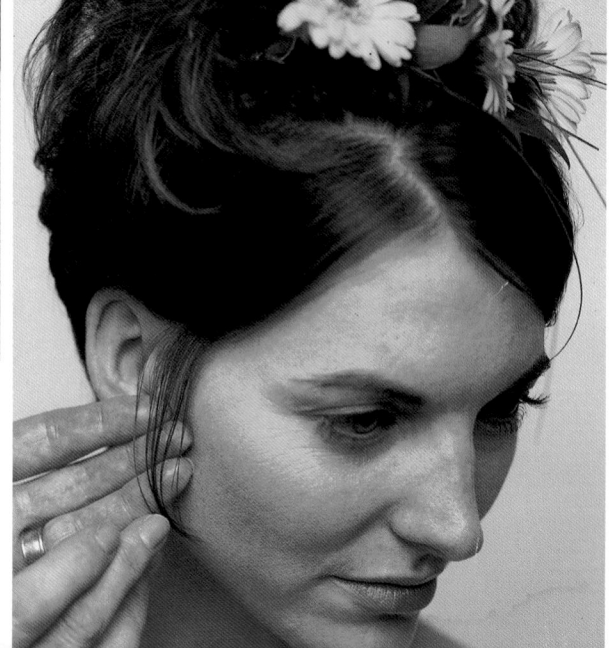

Flowers: The Flower Cellar

Opposite Dress: Kesté by Myring Kesterton

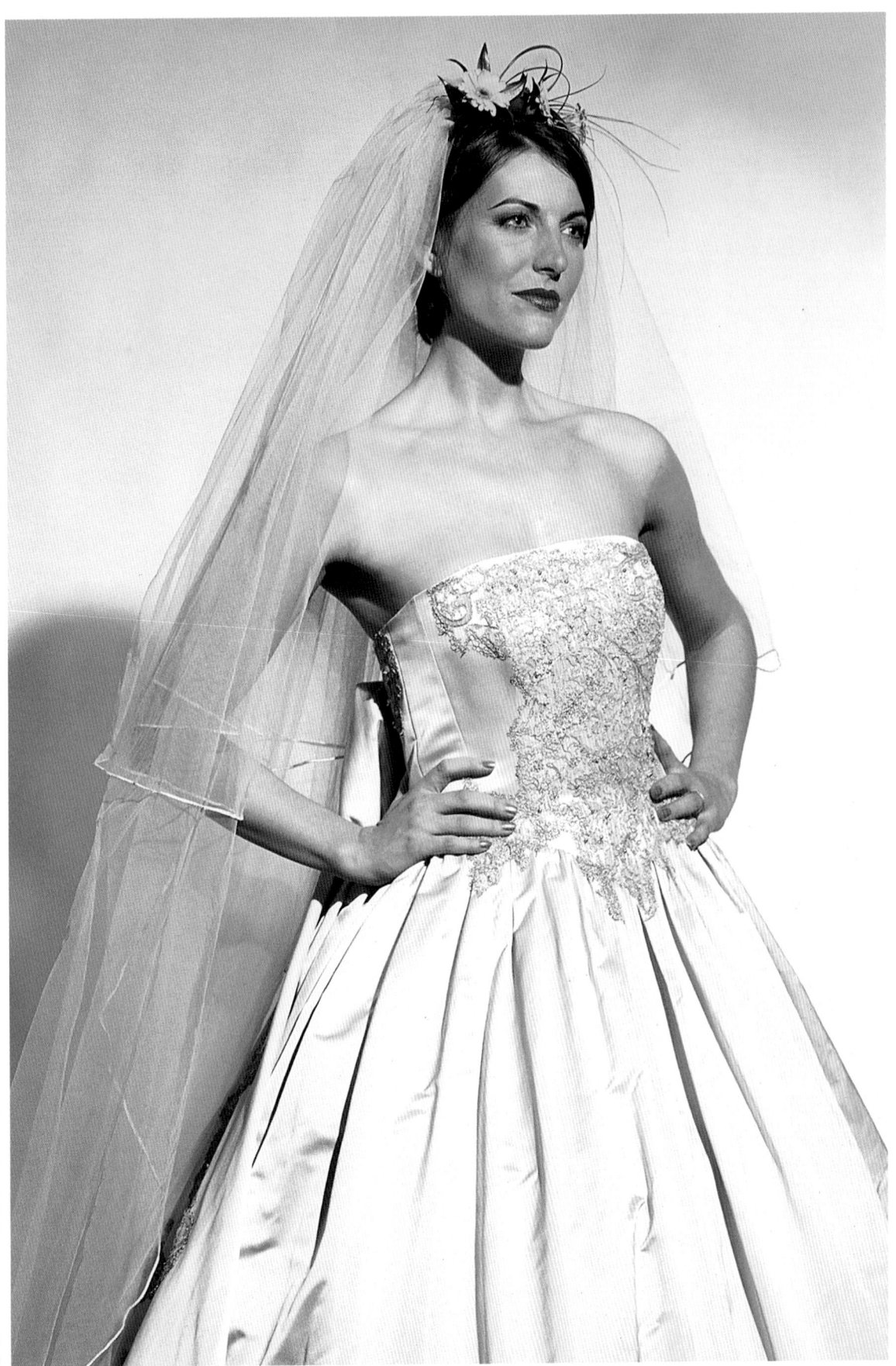

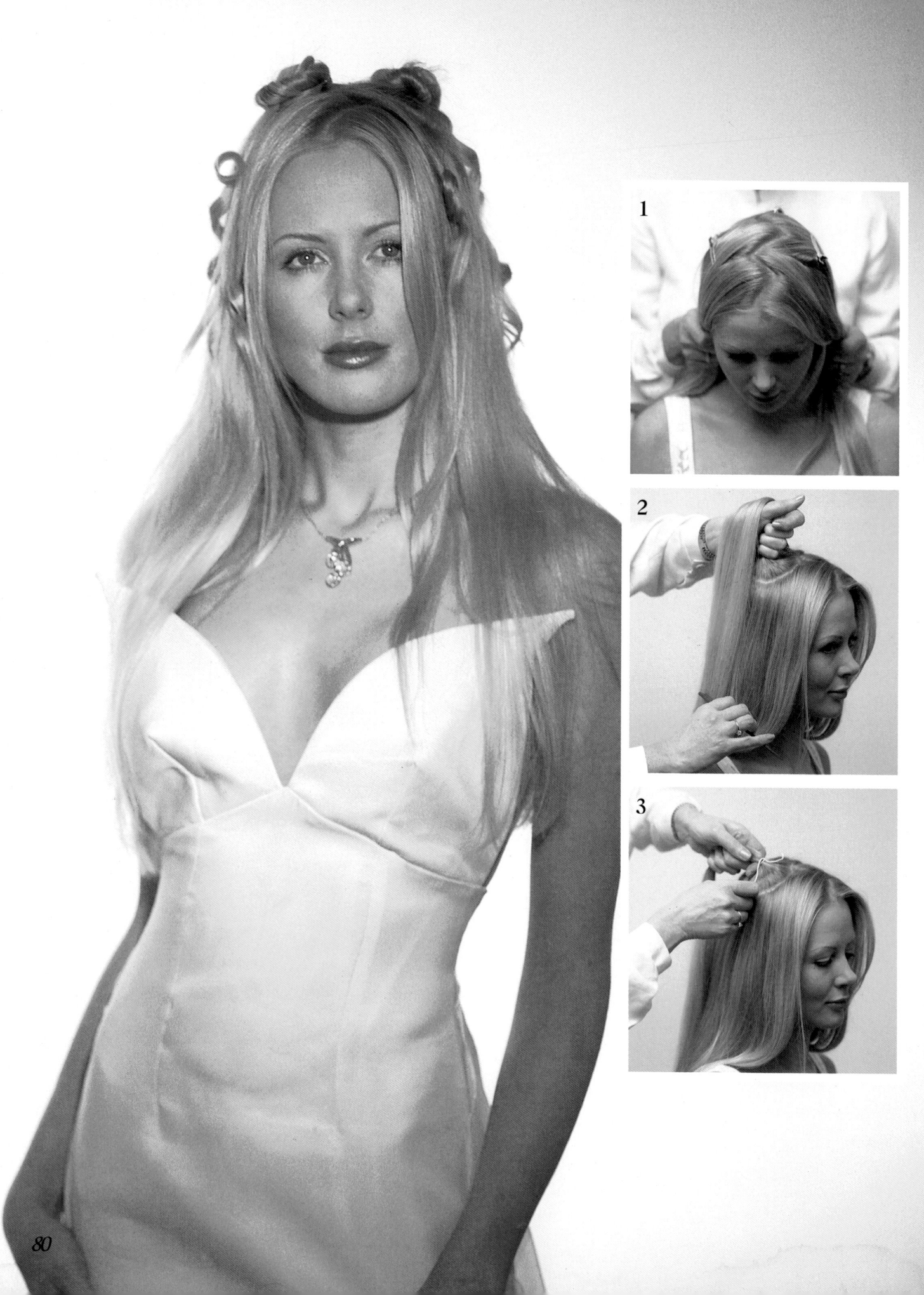

TULIP

1 Part hair in a zig-zag from forehead to crown.

— ✱ —

2 Take a section of hair, in a circle, from zig-zag parting and hold with hand.

— ✱ —

3 Secure section using dressmaking elastic.

— ✱ —

4 Take two more circular sections in same way – picture shows top view.

— ✱ —

5 Back view – the central section of hair has been lightly twisted to show partings clearly.

— ✱ —

6 Take the central back section and twist half way down length.

— ✱ —

7 The twist will begin to double back on itself and form a coil.

— ✱ —

8 Grip coil in place, leaving ends to fall free.

— ✱ —

9 Twist other two sections of hair in same way – picture shows all three coils completed.

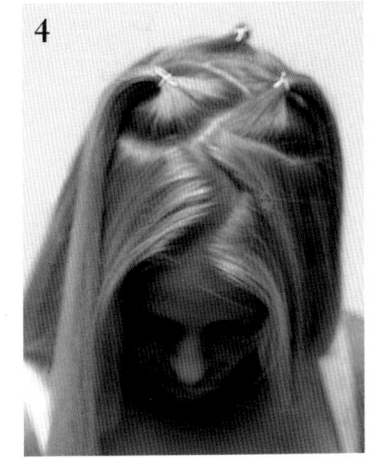

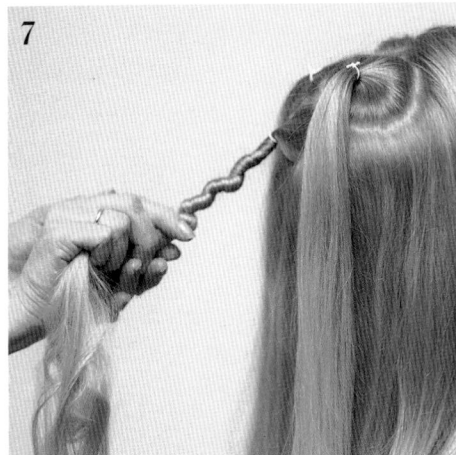

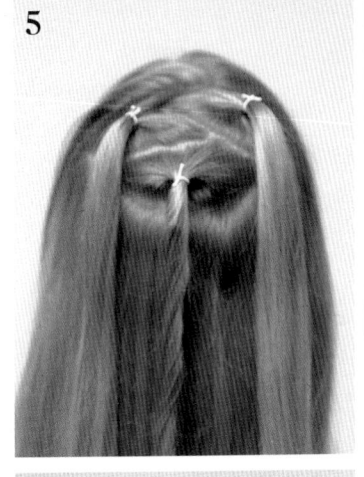

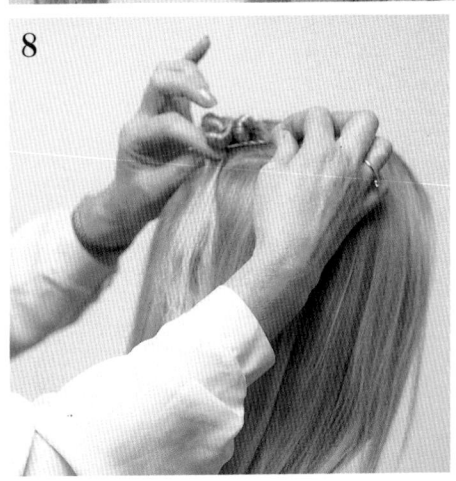

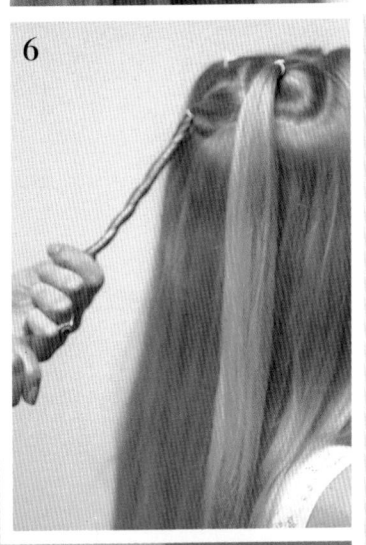

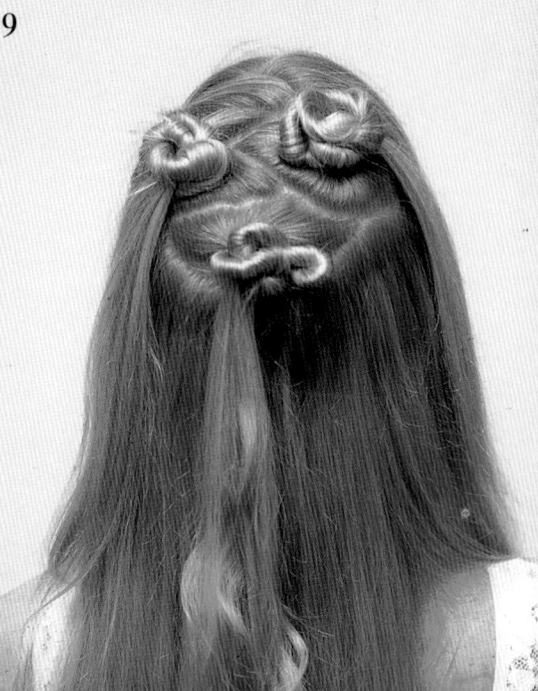

10 Divide free ends of one coiled section into three and randomly curl using tongs. Do not tong the entire section, just part, as shown, to achieve this texture mix.

——— ✳ ———

11 Repeat for other coiled sections.

——— ✳ ———

12 Take a small section of hair from side and tie into a knot just a little way from roots.

——— ✳ ———

13 Shows completed back view.

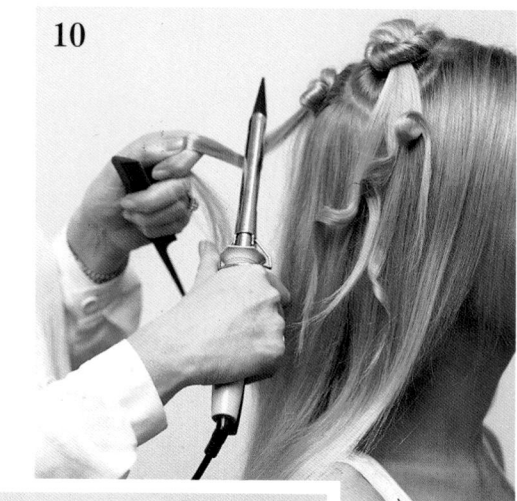

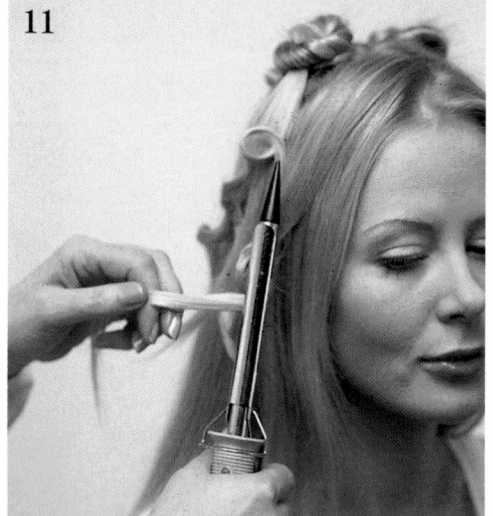

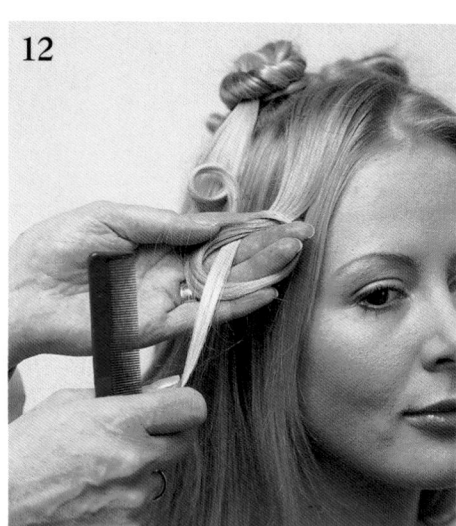

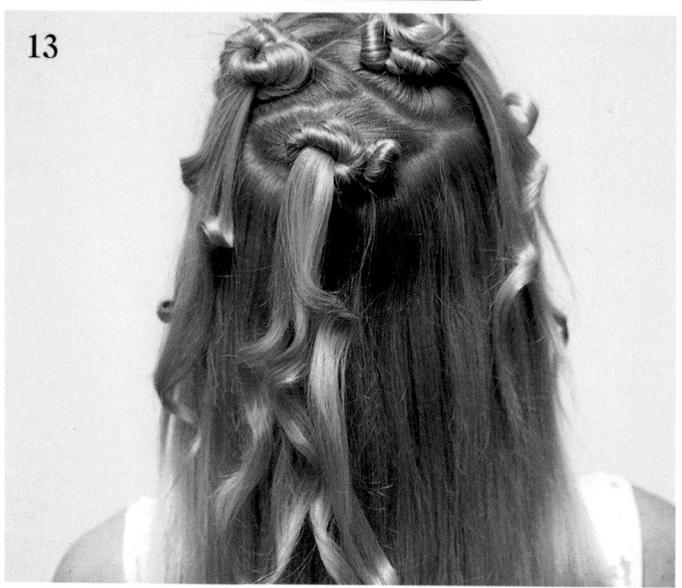

✳ ————————— ✳

𝒯IP

A light mist of spray shine will add a lovely shimmery gloss to this style.

✳ ————————— ✳

Opposite Dress: Kesté by Myring Kesterton

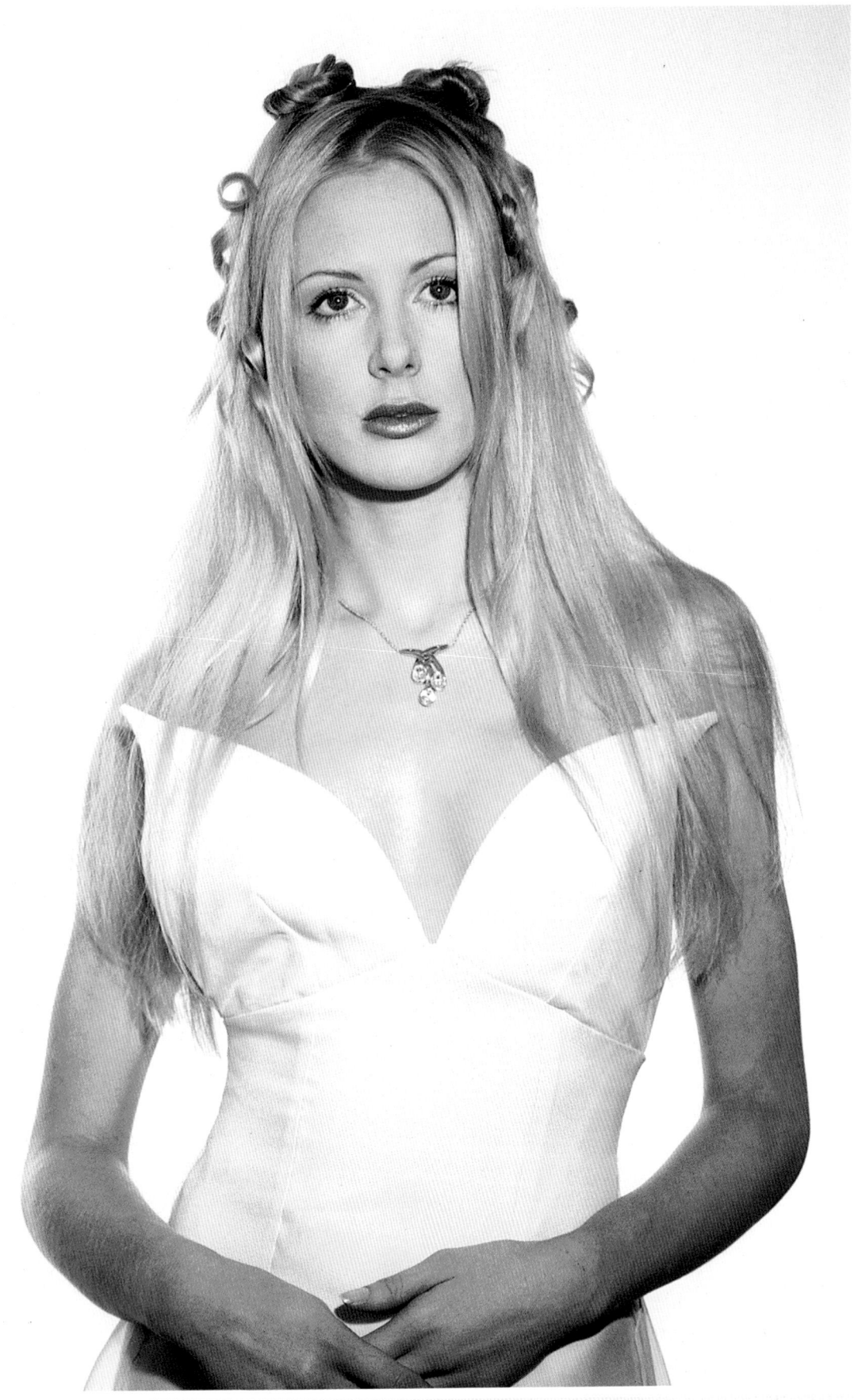

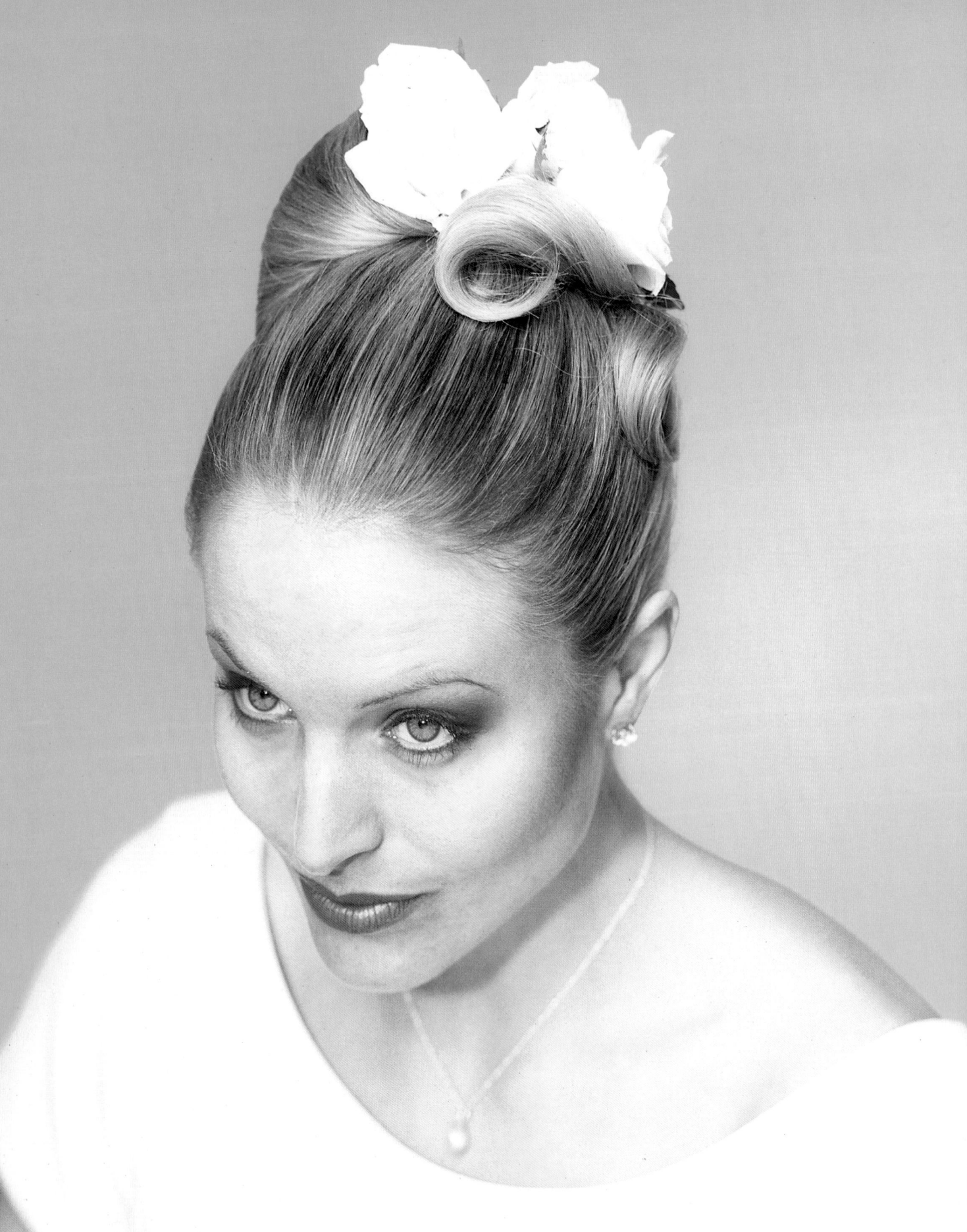

HELLENA

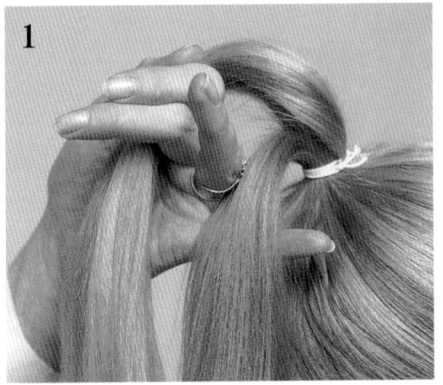

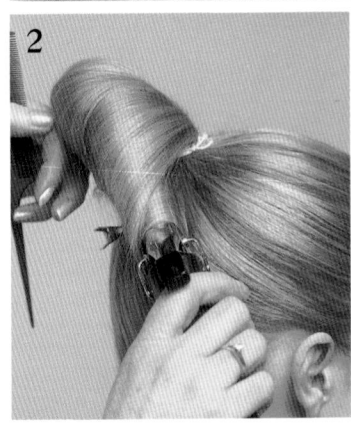

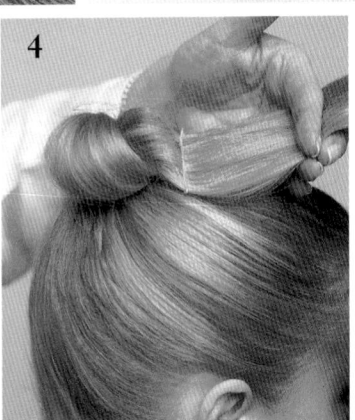

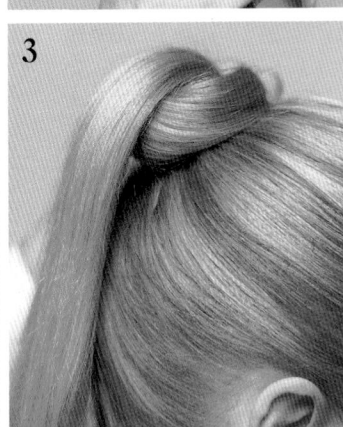

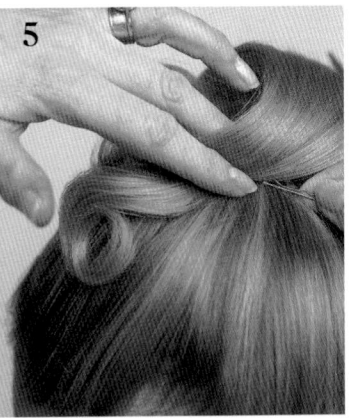

1 Smooth hair back into a high ponytail and secure with dressmaking elastic. Separate a quarter of the ponytail hair into a separate, smaller section.

———— ✳ ————

2 Tong each section of ponytail hair separately. Clipping one out of the way while you do the other.

———— ✳ ————

3 Take the small section of tonged hair and wrap round base of ponytail. Tuck ends in and grip in place.

———— ✳ ————

4 Take remaining larger section of hair and lightly backcomb. Flip forward and grip as shown.

———— ✳ ————

5 Curve back, allowing ends to form into a curl, and secure with grips.

———— ✳ ————

6 Position and grip flowers in place.

TIP

Try to use grips and pins that match the hair colour.

Opposite Dress: Classic Bridal Hire Collection

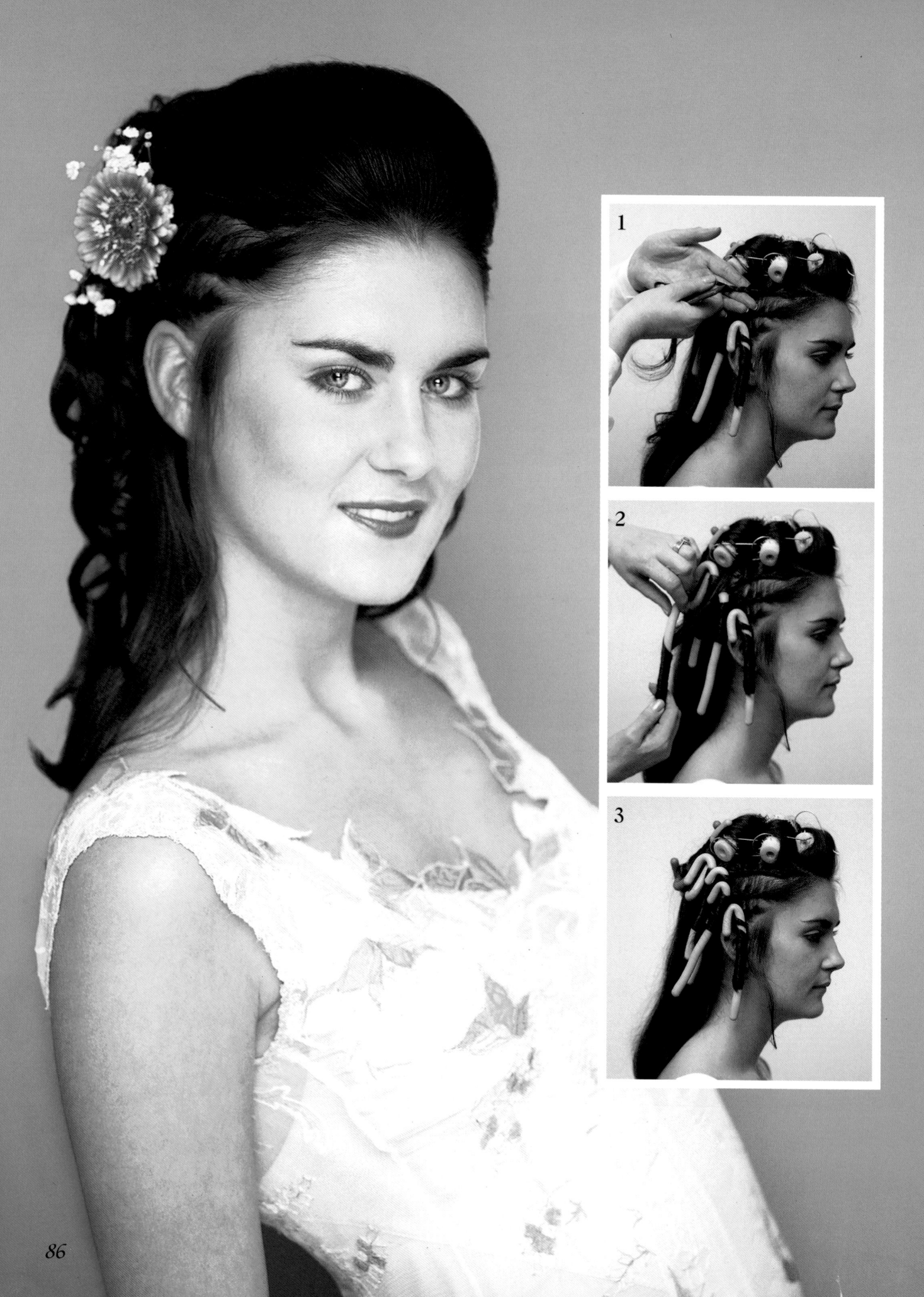

DAISY

1 Set crown hair on heated rollers straight back. Set back hair, from ear to ear, on hot sticks, working vertically. At one side, divide hair into three horizontal sections, leaving a tendril of hair to fall free. Start with lowest section and corn weave hair flat to head back towards ear. Secure by tying with cotton, then wind loose ends onto hot stick. Work on second section in same way.

———— ✻ ————

2 Work third section in same way, then repeat for other side.

———— ✻ ————

3 Shows completed pli.

———— ✻ ————

4 Blow-dry smooth the hair that was left out at the back.

———— ✻ ————

5 Unclip top of one hot stick and slide out of hair, keeping ringlet intact.

———— ✻ ————

6 Separate hair of ringlet into tendrils.

———— ✻ ————

7 Shows all hot sticks removed and hair cascading in tendrils.

———— ✻ ————

8 Remove heated rollers, except front one.

———— ✻ ————

9 Lightly backcomb crown hair at roots.

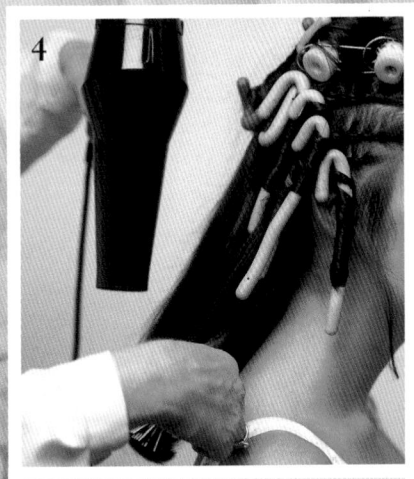

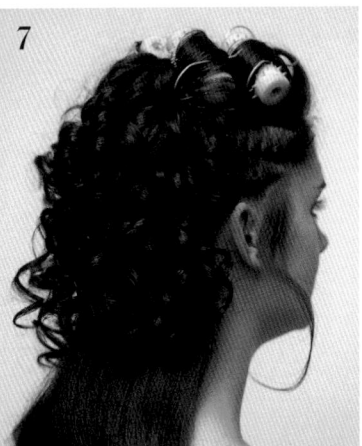

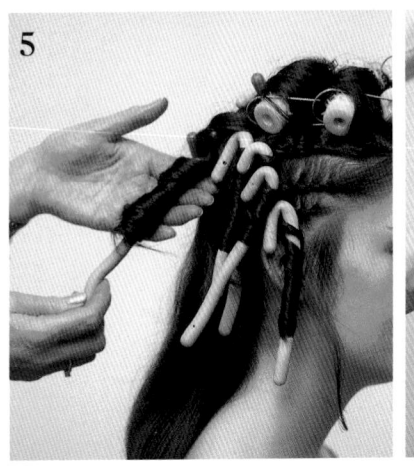

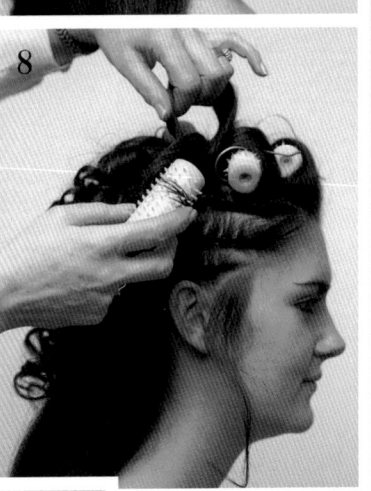

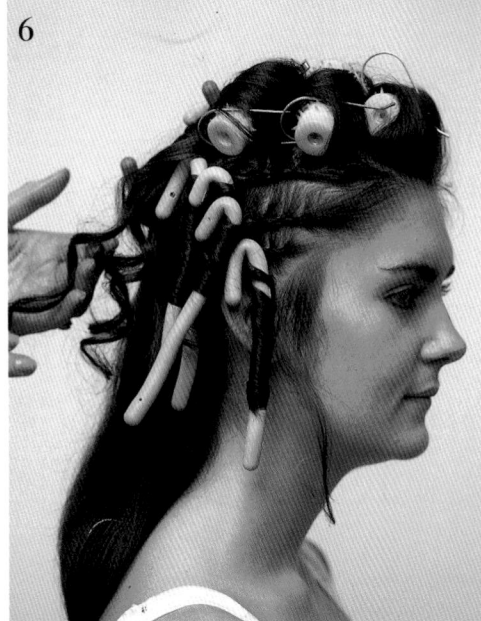

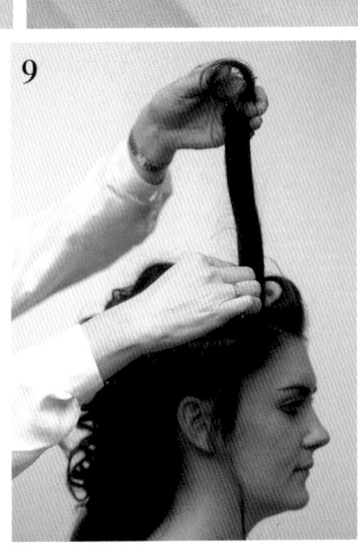

DAISY

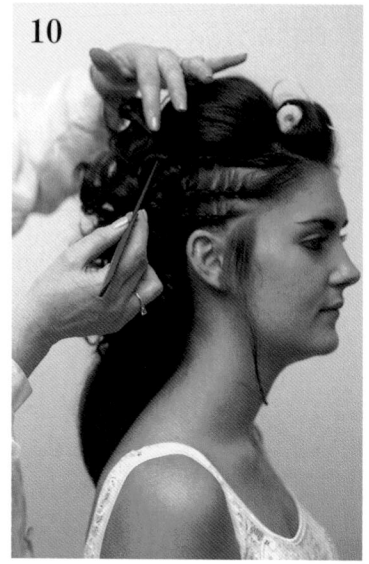

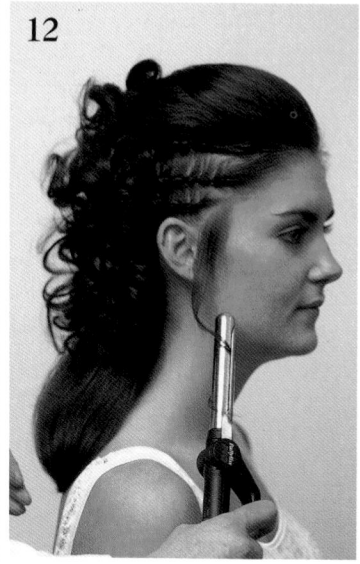

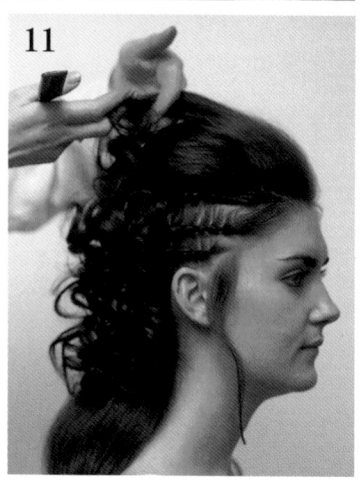

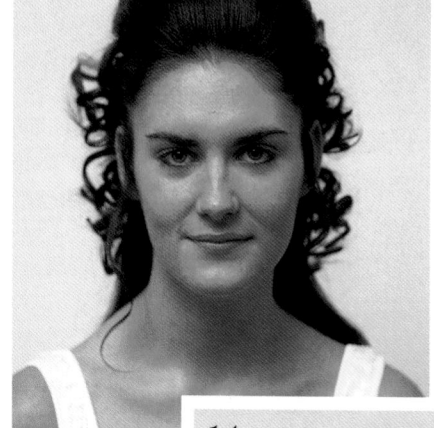

10 Smooth over and pin at top of ringlets.

———— ✳ ————

11 Remove remaining heated roller, lightly backcomb hair at roots and smooth over and clip in same way.

———— ✳ ————

12 Tong side tendrils.

———— ✳ ————

13 Shows completed front view.

———— ✳ ————

14 Shows completed side view.

TIP

For an even firmer set, use a dryer with a diffuser attachment set on a low heat/speed setting to further dry the hair. Allow hair to cool completely before removing rollers and hot sticks and styling as illustrated.

Opposite Dress: Kesté by Myring Kesterton

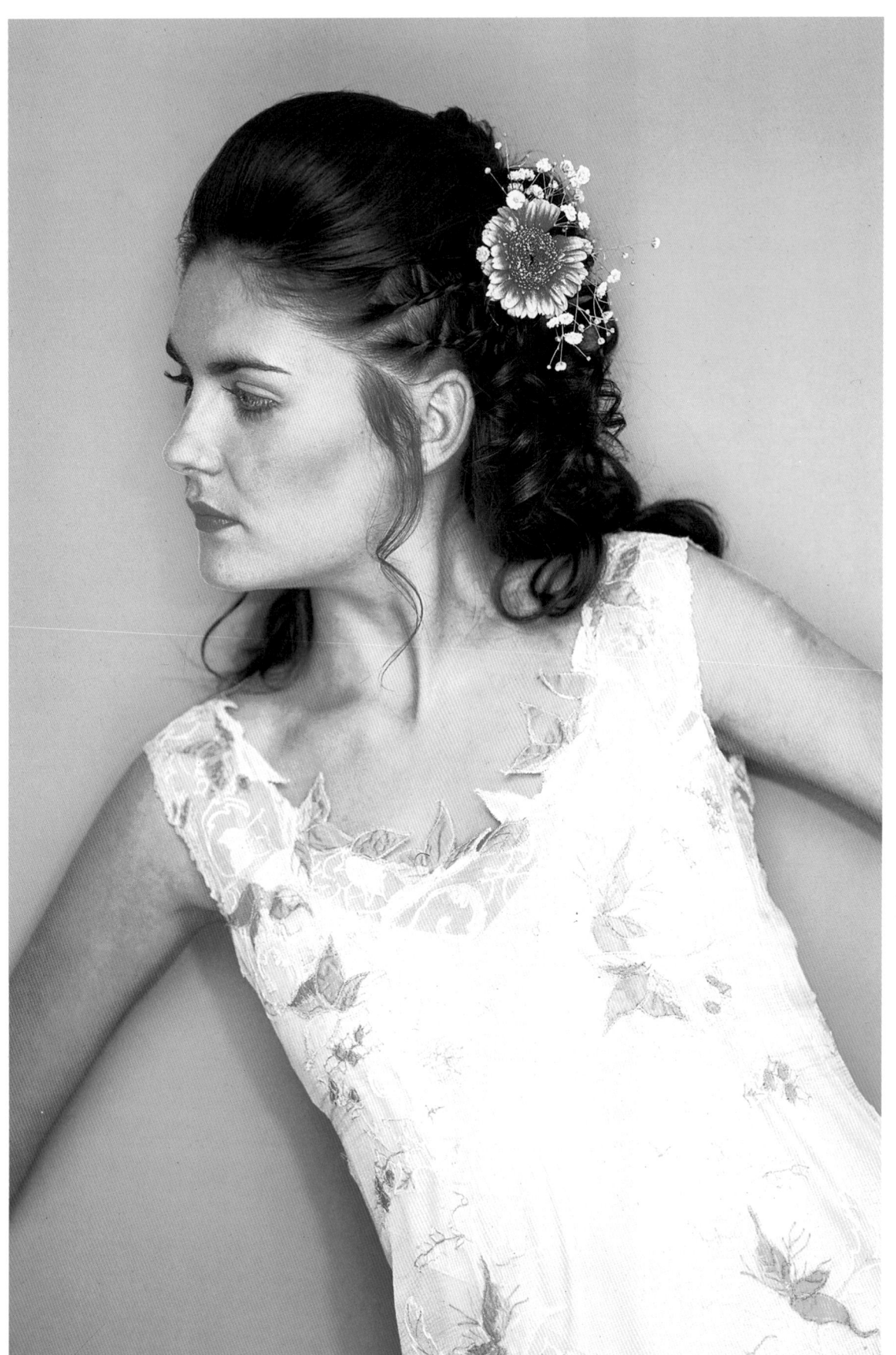

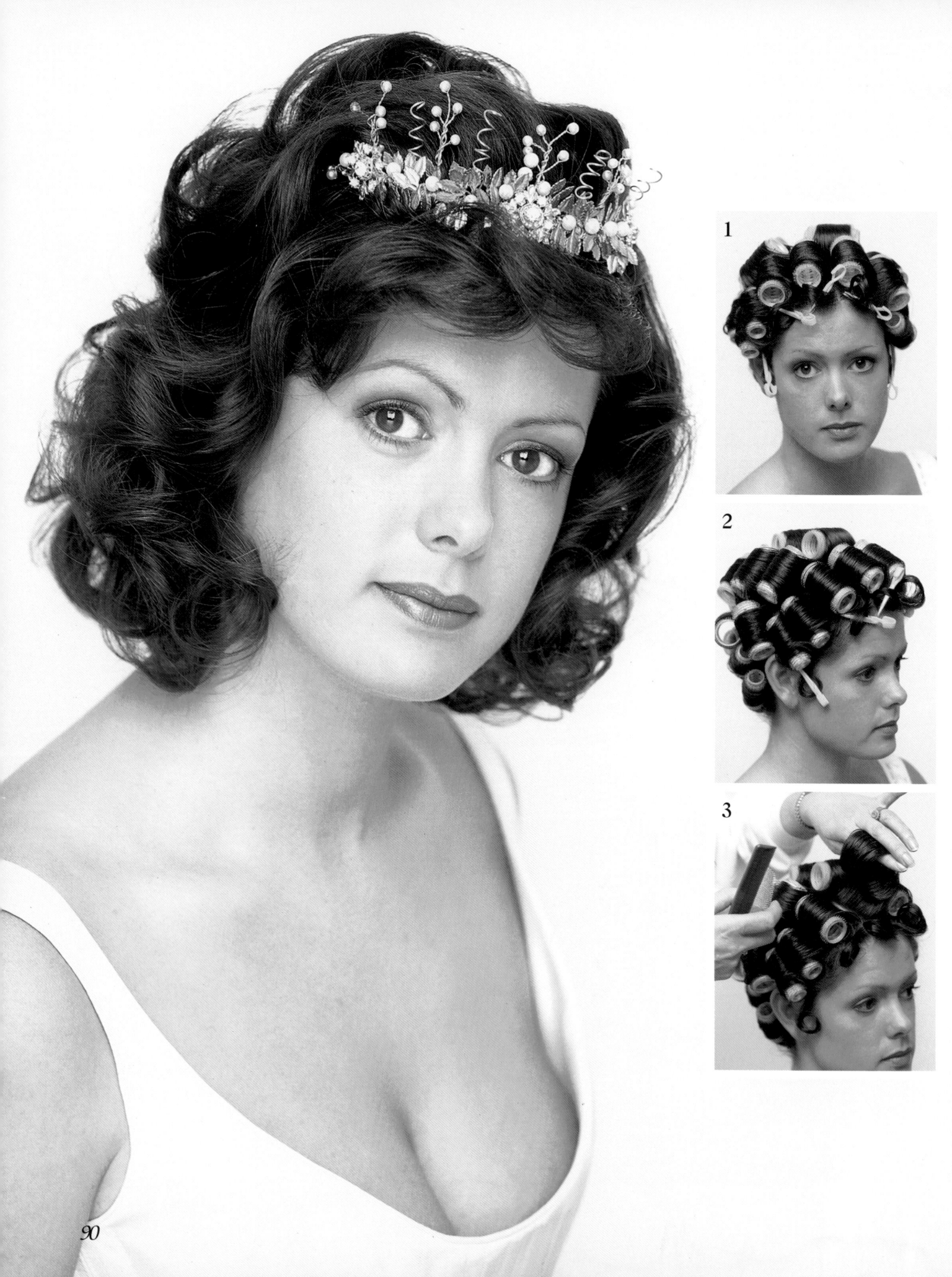

GYPSY

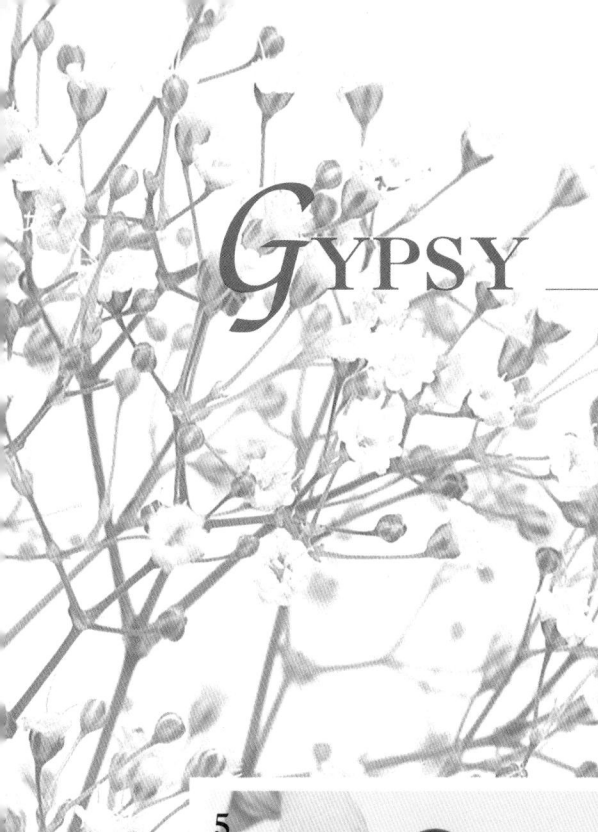

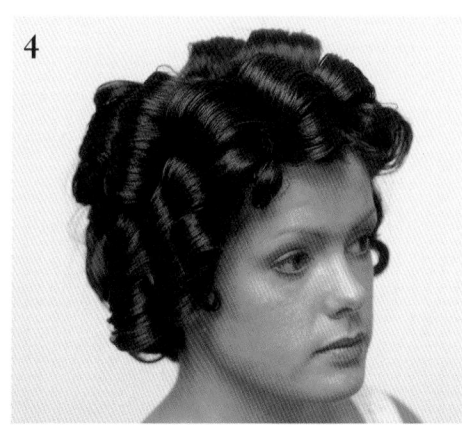

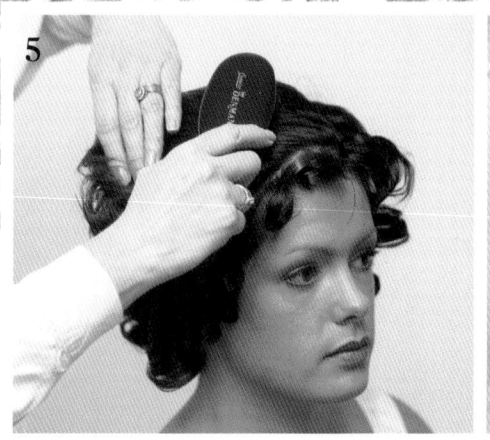

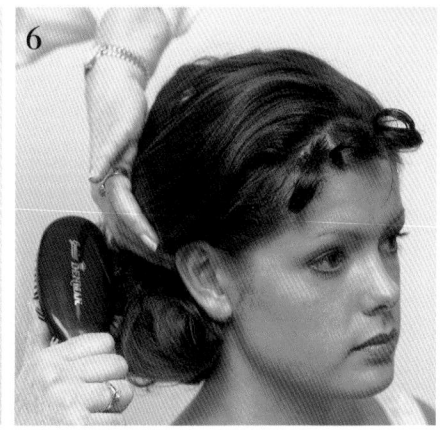

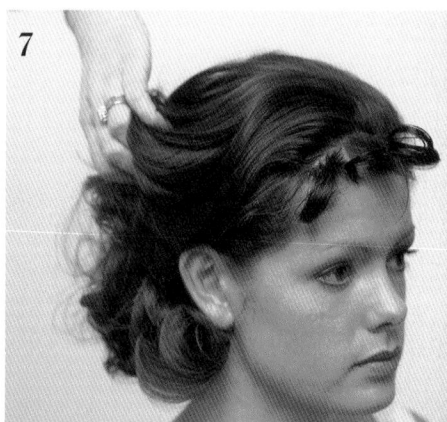

1 Set partially dried hair on self-fixing rollers – picture shows completed front view.

———— ✳ ————

2 Shows completed side view of pli with fringe and side hair set in barrel pin curls.

3 Hood dry. When hair is completely cold, remove rollers.

———— ✳ ————

4 Shows all rollers removed.

———— ✳ ————

5 Start smoothing hair from front, using a bristle brush.

———— ✳ ————

6 Brush right through to ends, flicking hair out.

———— ✳ ————

7 Mist with hairspray while lifting with fingers to give volume and texture.

———— ✳ ————

8 Position head-dress and grip in place, then comb fringe.

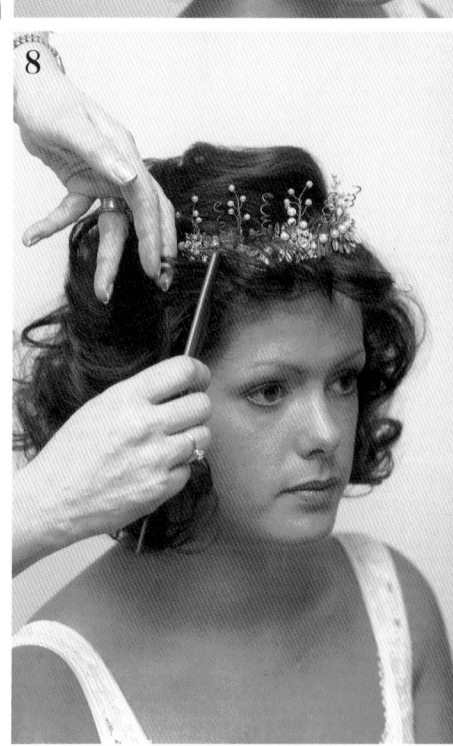

TIP

Use self-fixing rollers with a heat-retaining metallic band – they give a firmer, longer-lasting set.

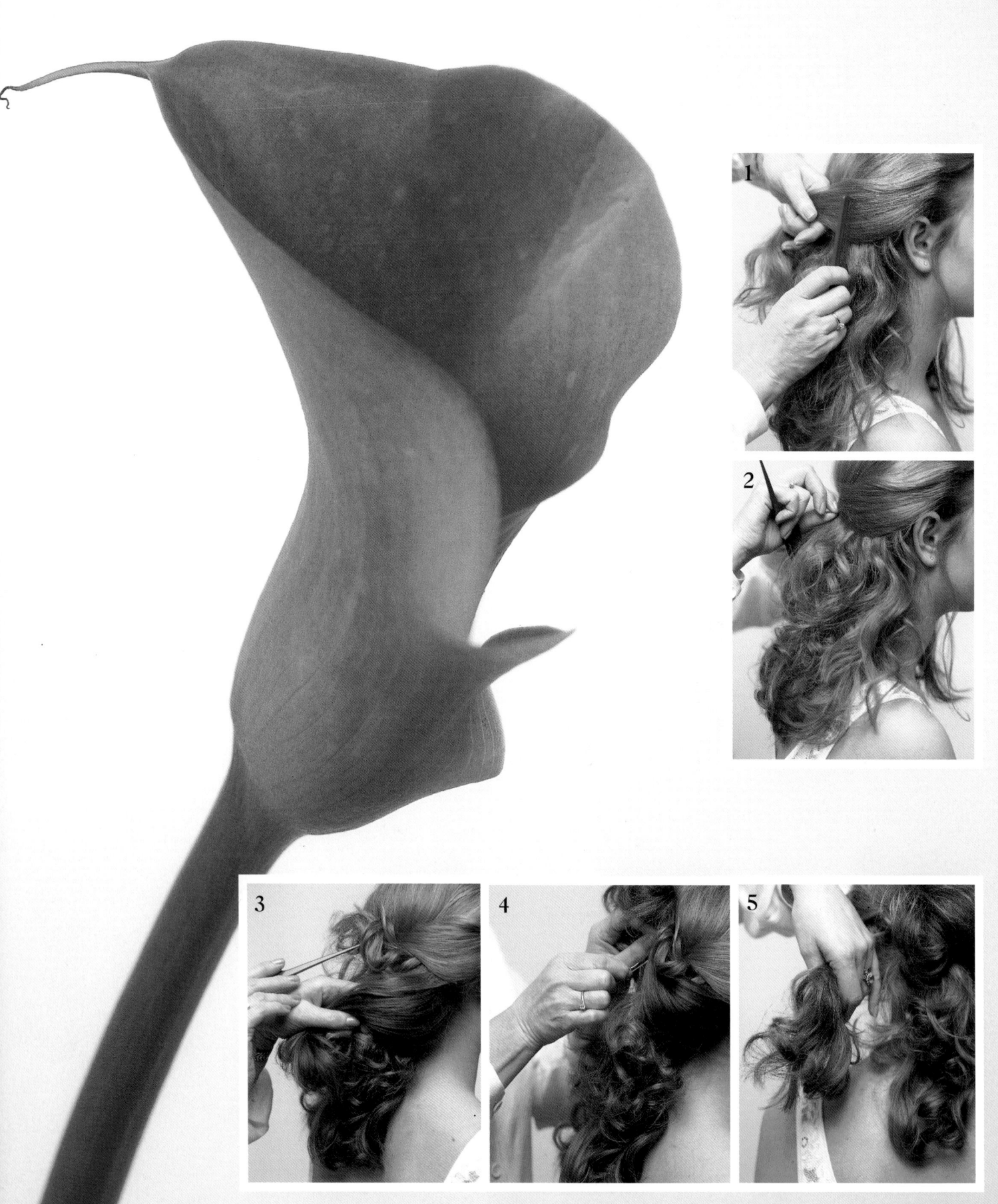

ARIES

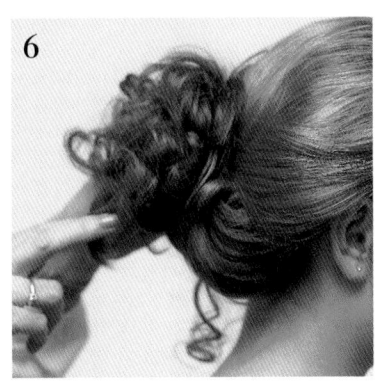
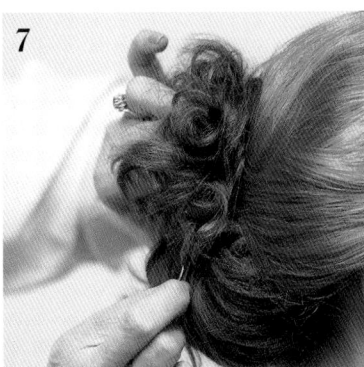

1 Take section from side and slightly twist to centre back.

———— ✳ ————

2 Secure with a grip.

———— ✳ ————

3 Repeat for other side. Divide lower section into three, leaving a few curls out at centre back.

———— ✳ ————

4 Roll one side section of hair from nape and secure at centre back with a grip.

———— ✳ ————

5 Repeat for other side.

———— ✳ ————

6 Scoop up remaining centre section and secure with grips.

———— ✳ ————

7 Gently dress curls to give full and natural movement.

TIP

Mist finished hairstyle with a light hold product so that when hair is let down, it will fall into soft, tumbling waves and won't feel sticky.

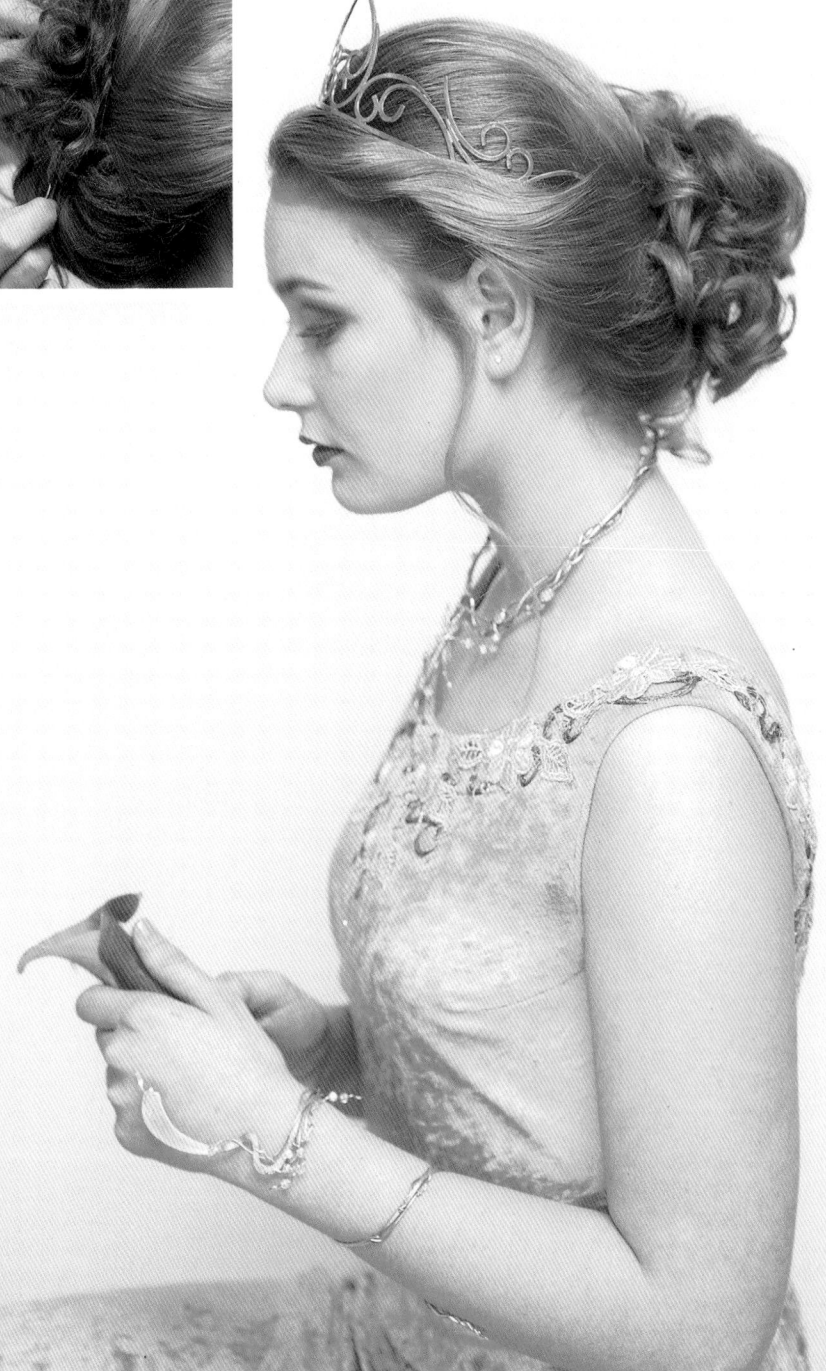

Dress and jewellery: Kesté by Myring Kesterton
Tiara: Classics Bridal Hire Collection

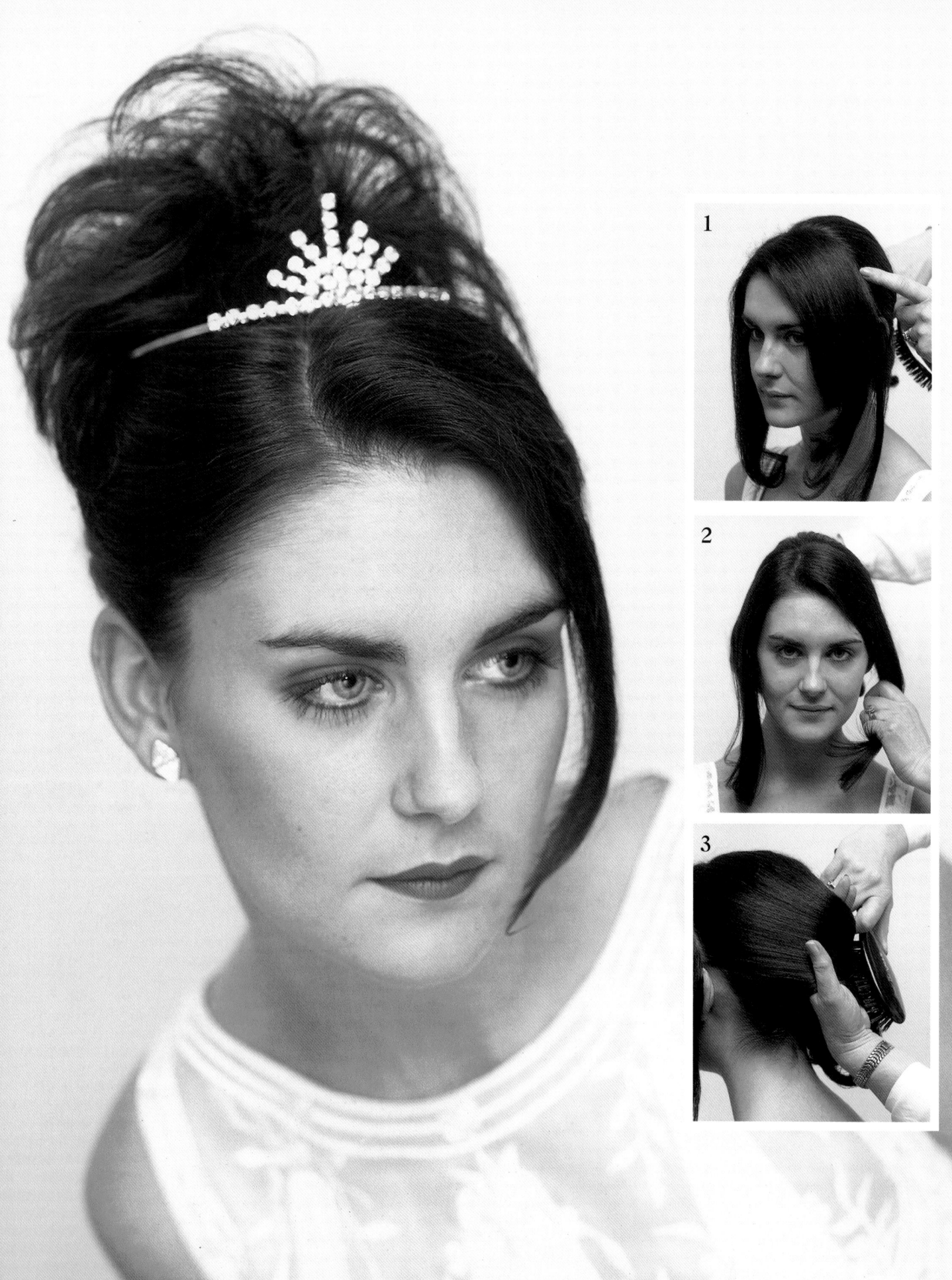

MIMOSA

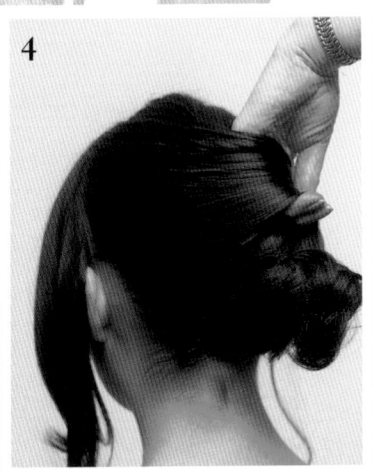

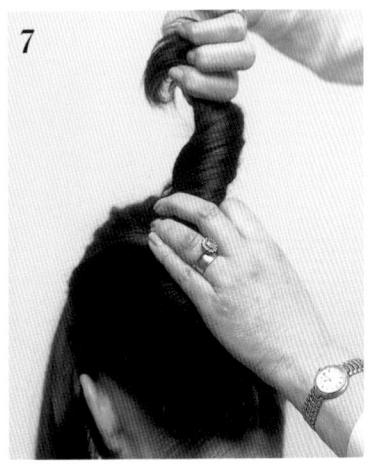

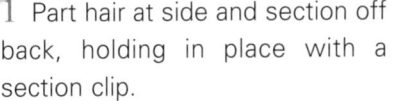

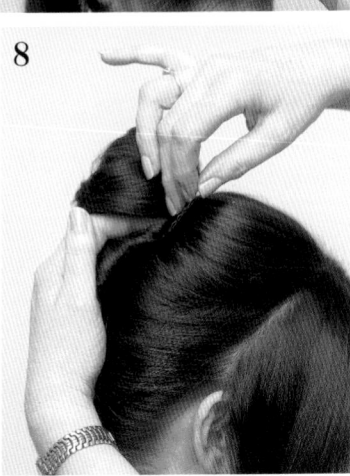

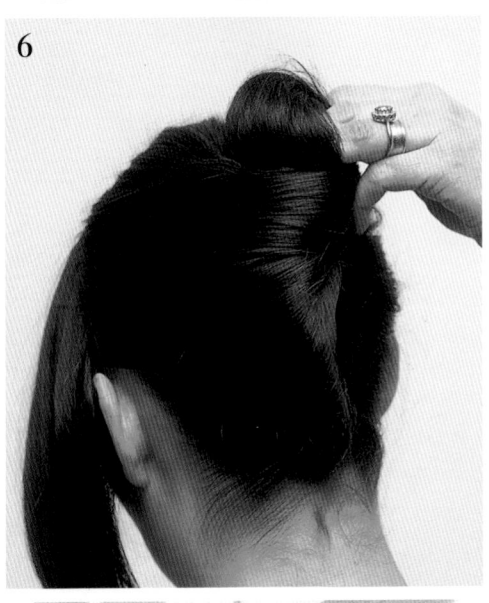

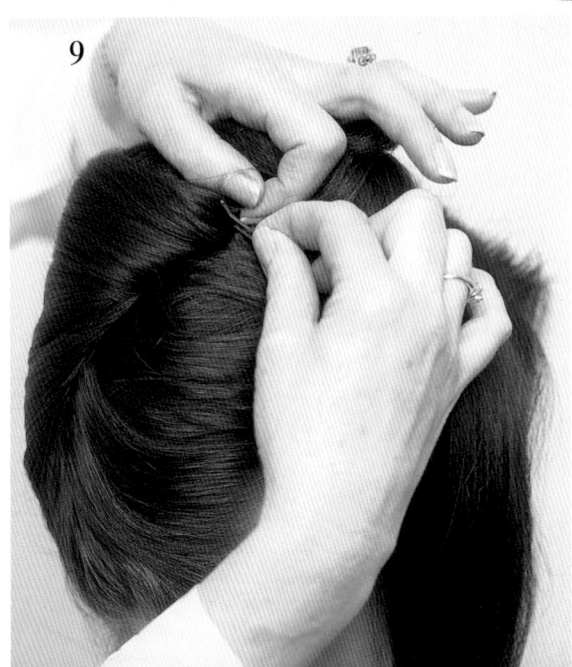

1 Part hair at side and section off back, holding in place with a section clip.

———✳———

2 Shows front view of sectioning.

———✳———

3 Unclip back section and use a bristle brush to smooth hair.

———✳———

4 Twist hair around fingers as if tying a knot.

———✳———

5 Pull knot up ...

———✳———

6 ... and through.

———✳———

7 Pull out ends and twist.

———✳———

8 Secure with grip inserted vertically down twisted section.

———✳———

9 Now grip horizontally.

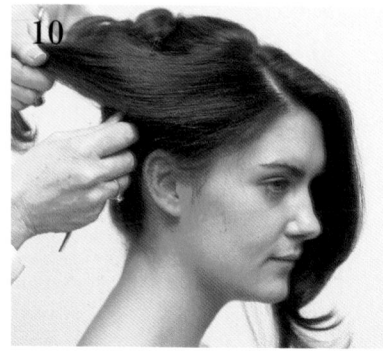

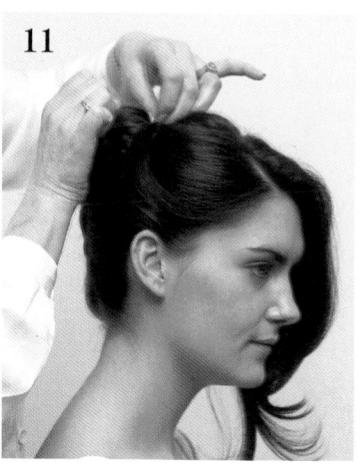

10 Bring up one section of side hair and lightly backcomb.

———— ✳ ————

11 Smooth this hair to crown, curving into place and leaving ends free. Grip in place.

———— ✳ ————

12 Take other side, separate out a small section and leave to fall free and curve onto face. Backcomb the main section and smooth over, taking ends to crown, curving into place and allowing ends to form a tuft. Grip into place.

———— ✳ ————

13 Backcomb tuft of hair from the knot, leaving the two ends that were taken from the sides free.

———— ✳ ————

14 Shows back view with ends backcombed.

———— ✳ ————

15 Finally, backcomb ends of curved hair that was left free and fan out.

———— ✳ ————

16 Push tiara into place and secure with a grip.

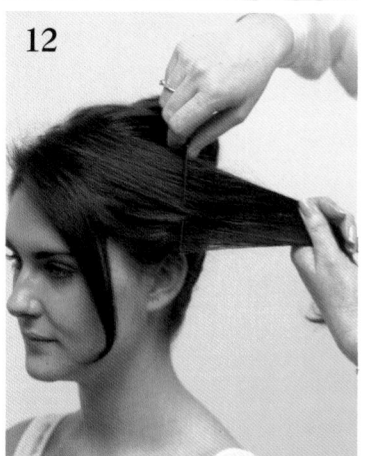

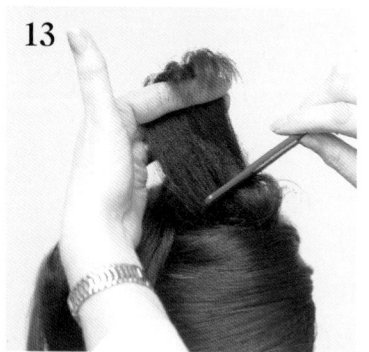

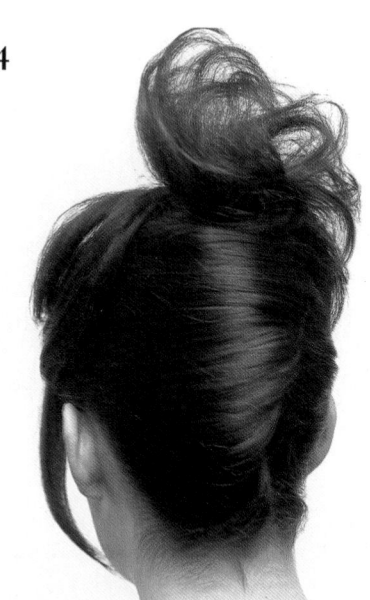

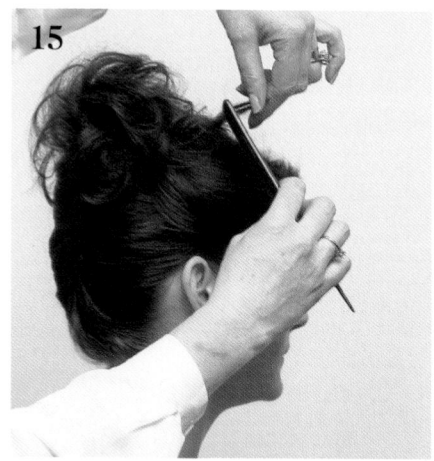

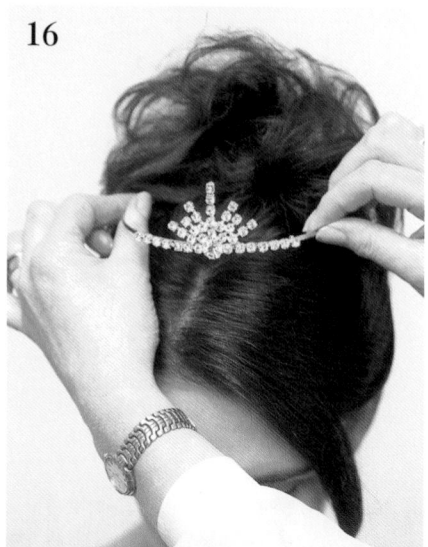

✳ ———————————— ✳

𝒯IP

This is a versatile style that is suitable for all types of head-dresses.

✳ ———————————— ✳

Opposite Dress and head-dress: Classics Bridal Hire Collection

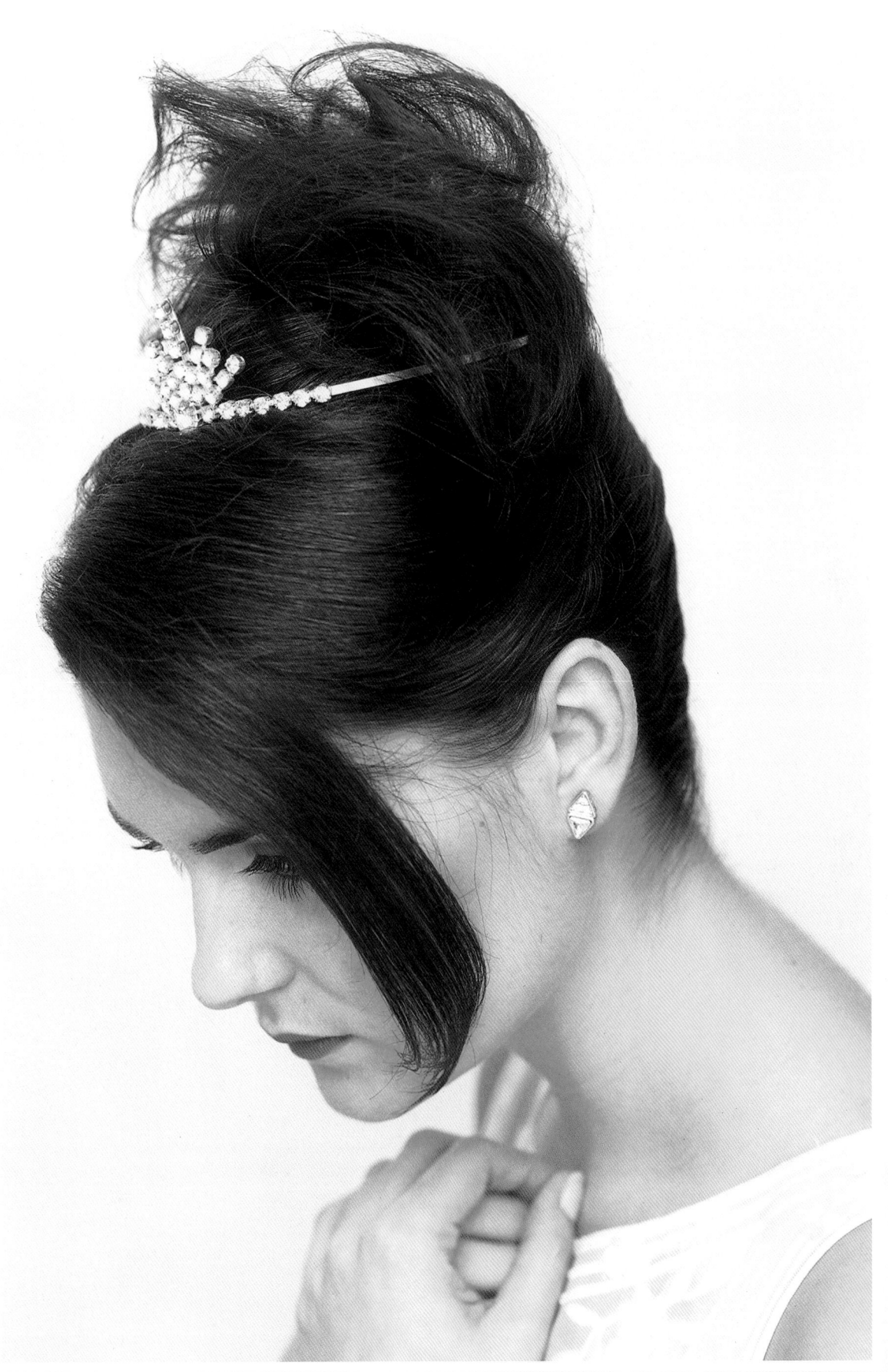

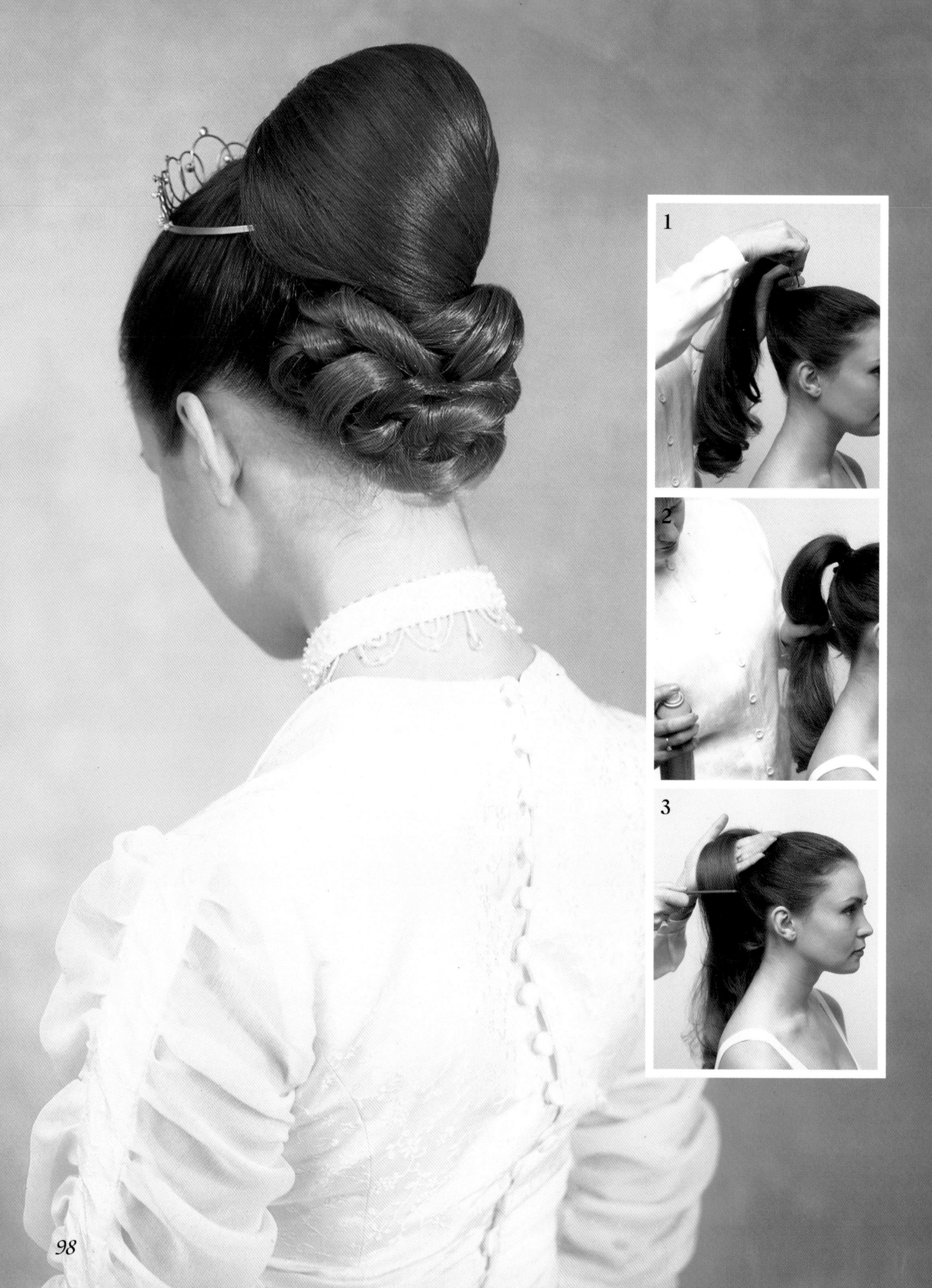

ROSE

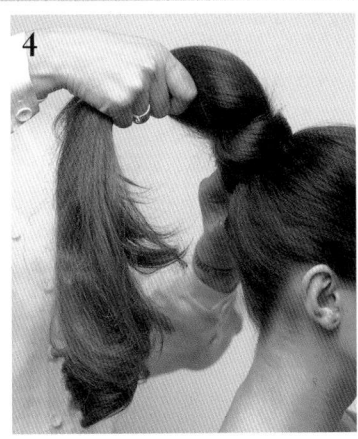

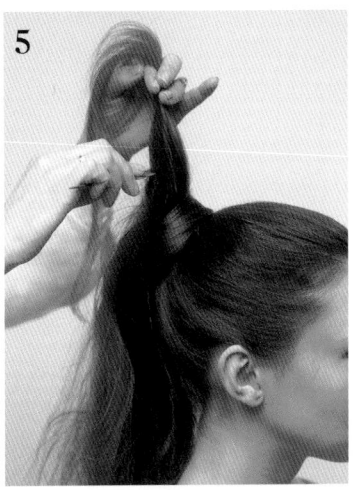

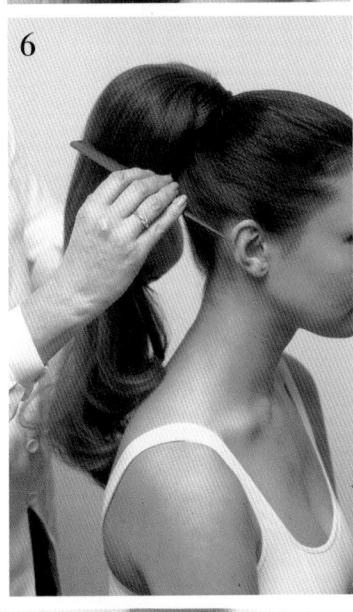

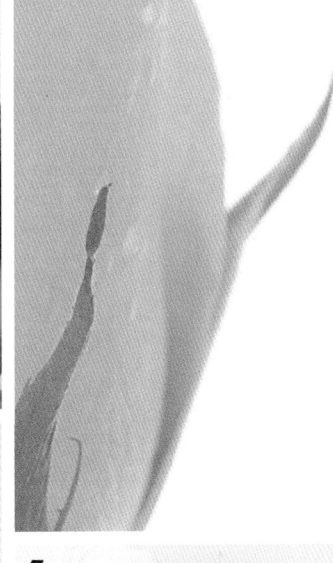

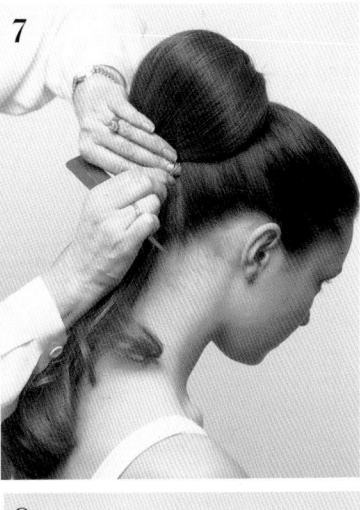

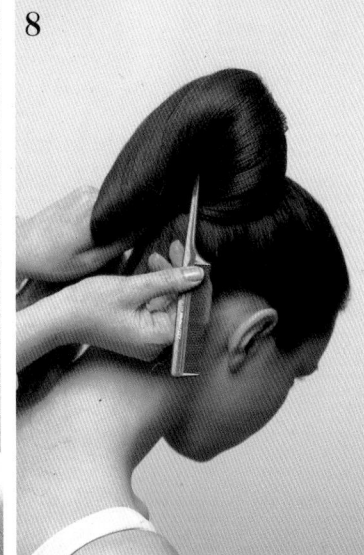

1 Smooth hair back to crown and secure in band.

———— ✳ ————

2 Mist with hairspray to smooth any frizzy ends.

———— ✳ ————

3 Take a small section of hair from underneath ponytail and comb smooth.

———— ✳ ————

4 Wrap this piece of hair round base of ponytail and grip underneath to secure.

———— ✳ ————

5 Take ponytail and backcomb at roots.

———— ✳ ————

6 Smooth top layer of hair.

———— ✳ ————

7 Grip into place.

———— ✳ ————

8 Clasp length of ponytail in one hand and twist slightly to one side, using end of tail comb to achieve shape.

———— ✳ ————

9 Secure with grips positioned vertically as shown.

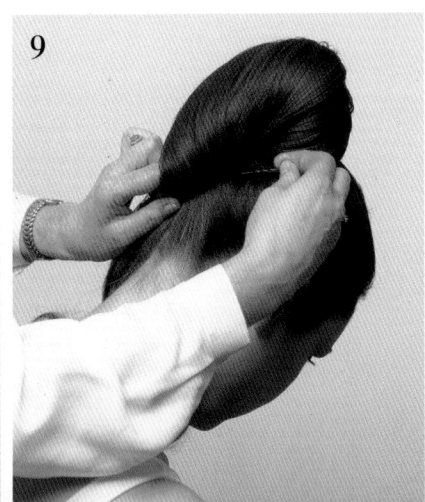

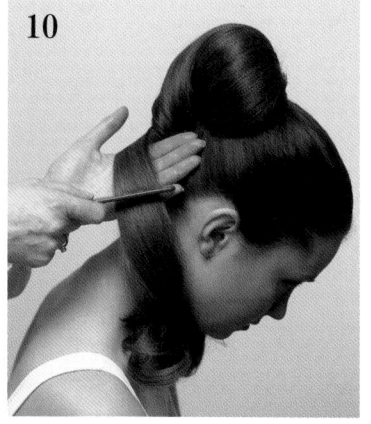

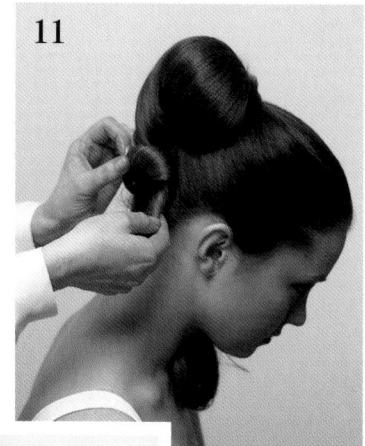

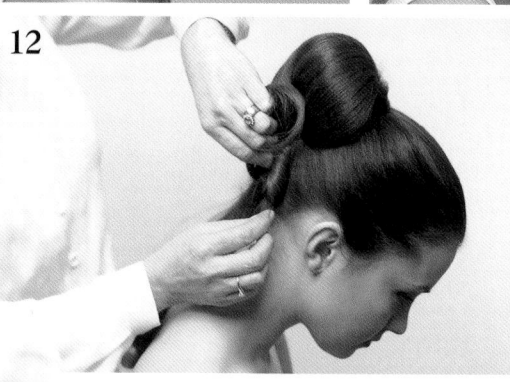

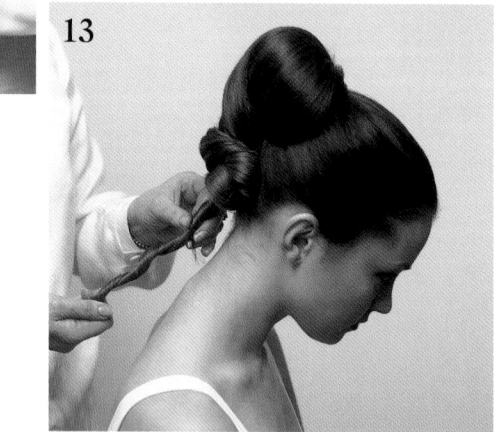

10 Divide remaining hair into two sections, comb one smooth.

———— ✳ ————

11 Twist this section until hair starts to double back on itself and form a curl.

———— ✳ ————

12 Secure with grips.

———— ✳ ————

13 Twist remaining section of hair and grip into place in same way.

———— ✳ ————

14 Shows back view. Add tiara and grip into place.

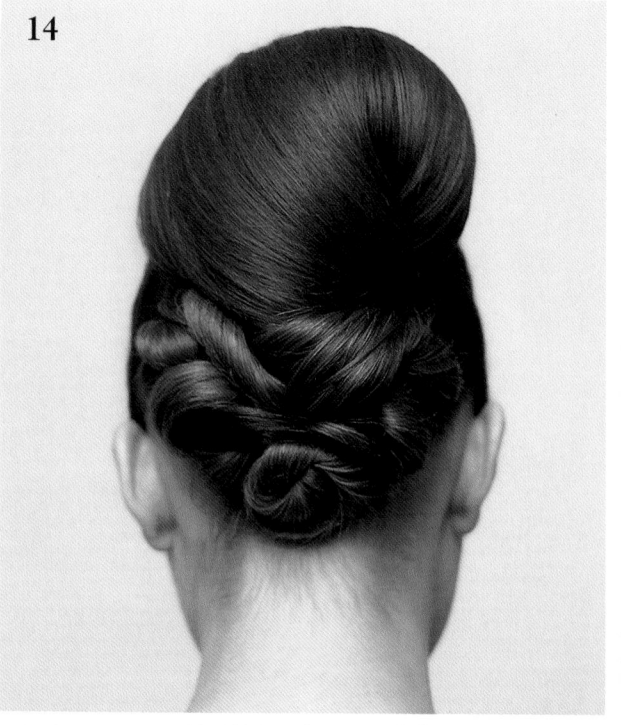

✳ ———————————— ✳

𝒯IP

When smoothing hair over, mist comb with hairspray to help slick in stray ends.

✳ ———————————— ✳

Opposite Dress, head-dress, and choker: Cocoa

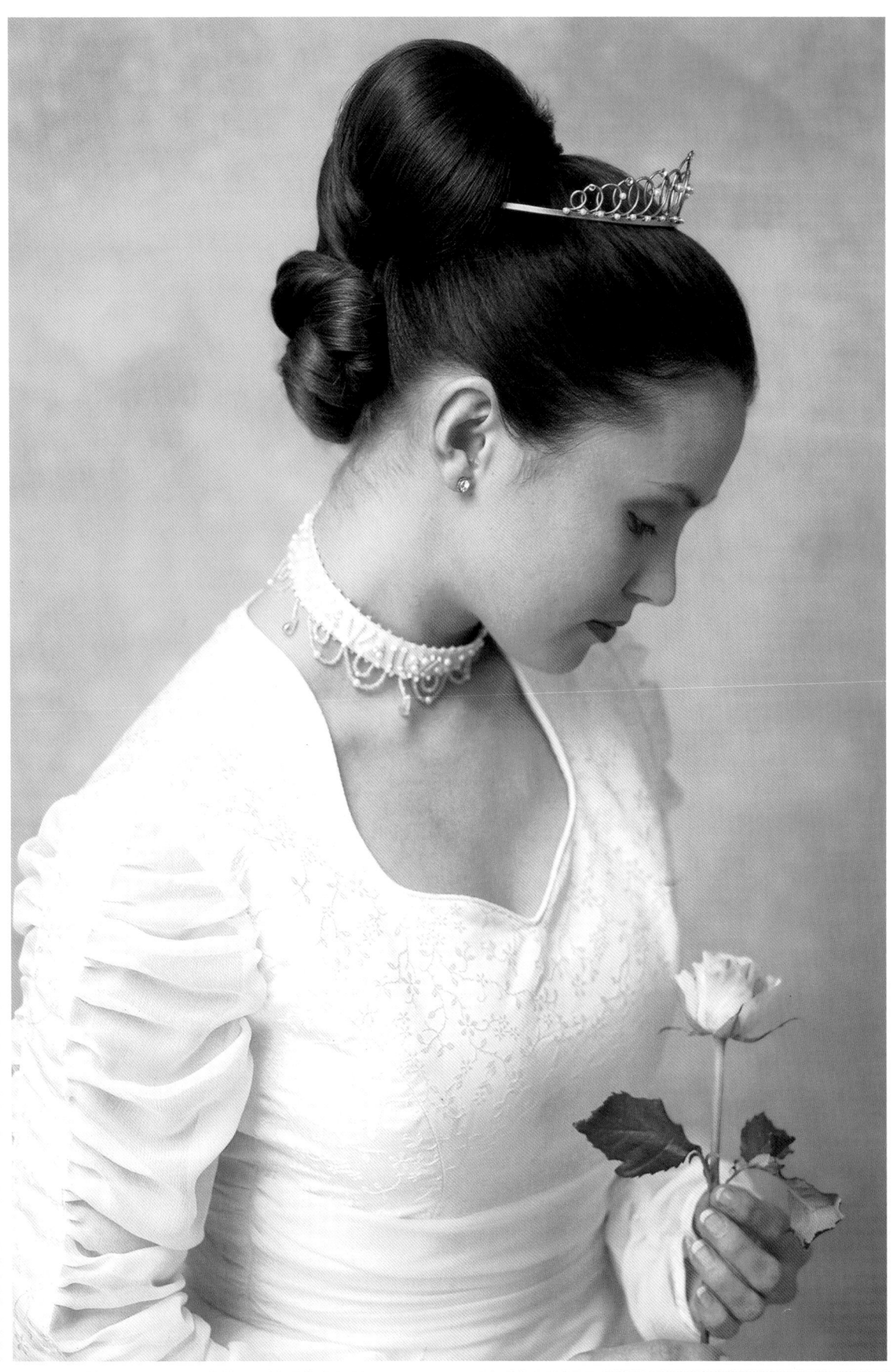

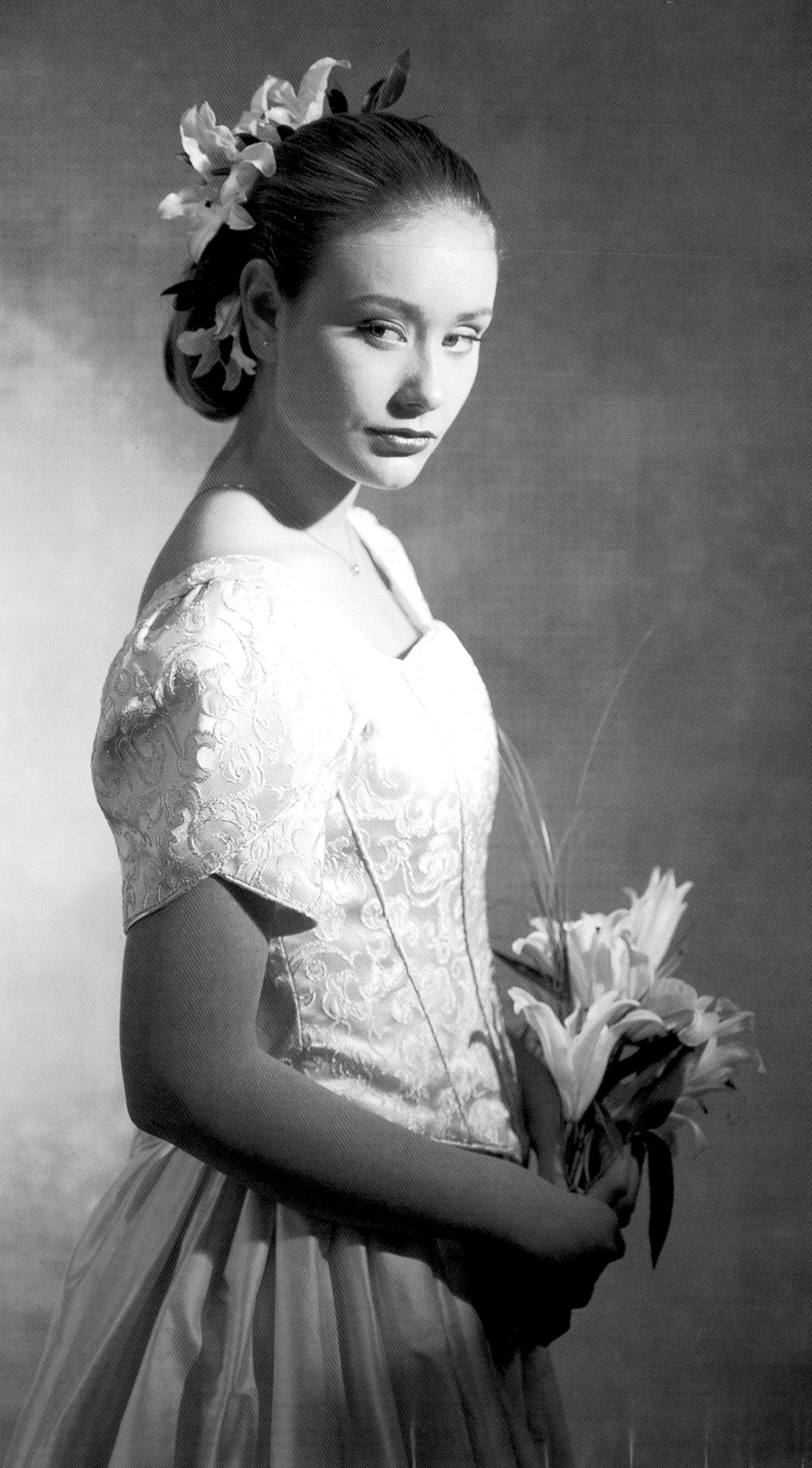

LILY

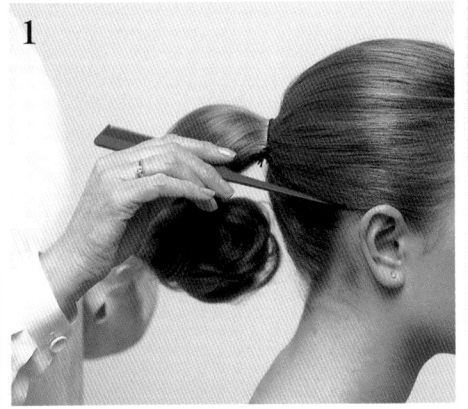

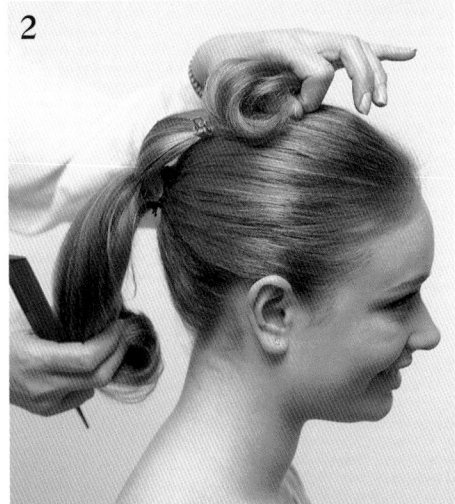

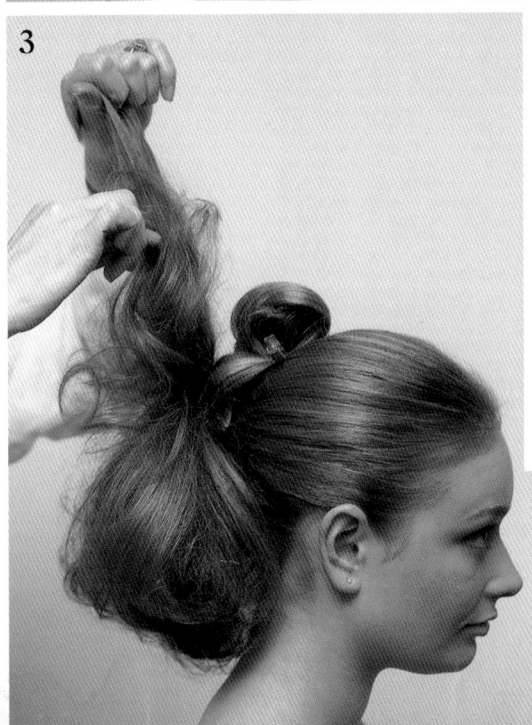

1 Smooth hair into a ponytail, making sure that base aligns with top of ear.

———— ✳ ————

2 Section off top third of ponytail and clip out of the way.

———— ✳ ————

3 Backcomb remaining hair – firmly at base of ponytail but lightly at ends. Mist with hairspray.

———— ✳ ————

4 Smooth ponytail using a tail comb.

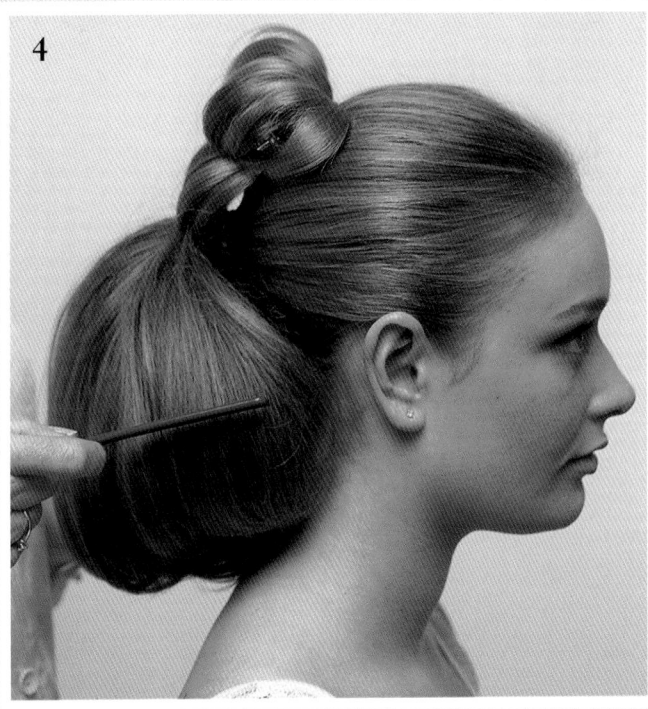

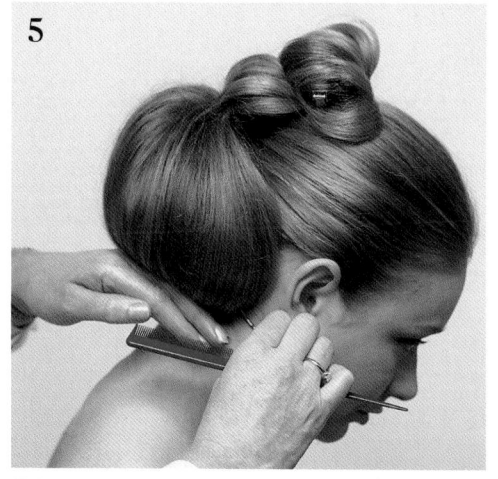

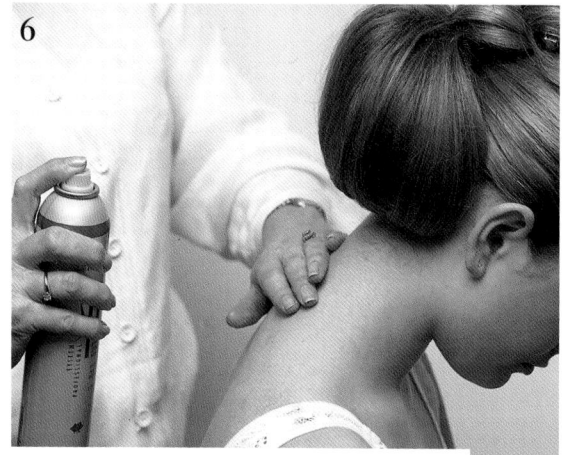

5 Tuck in ends and pin into place.

———— ✳ ————

6 Mist underneath with hairspray, making sure you use sufficient product to ensure a firm hold.

———— ✳ ————

7 Unclip reserved section of hair, then divide into three equal sections.

———— ✳ ————

8 Lightly backcomb centre section.

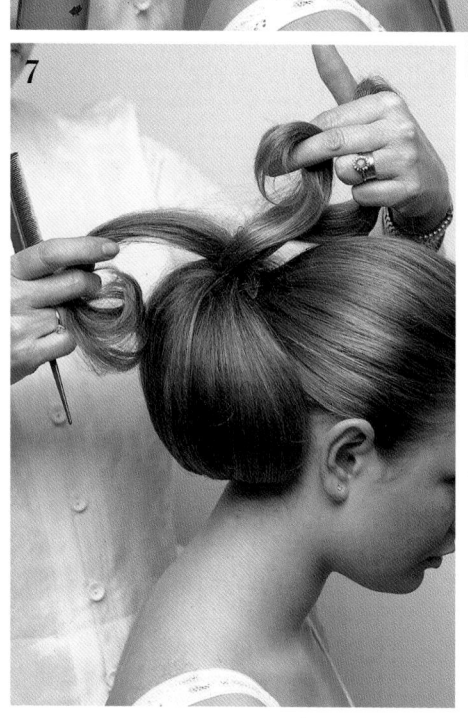

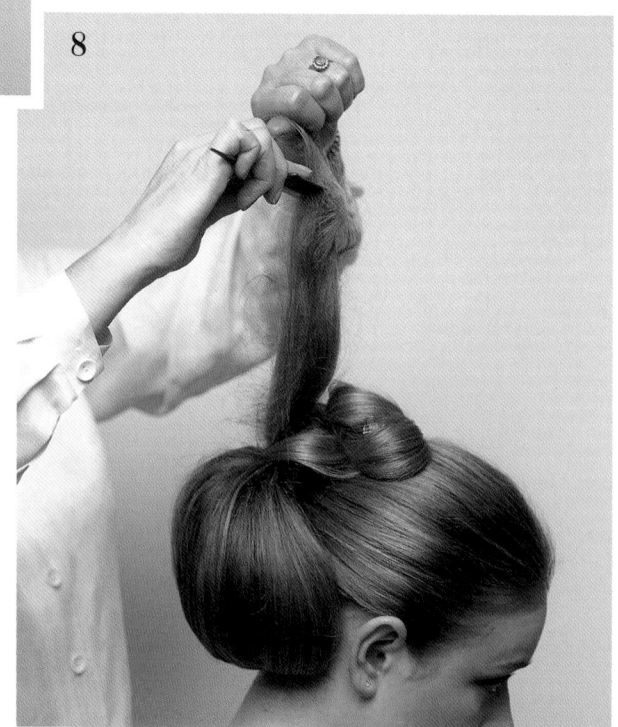

9 Hold section upwards and insert two grips, crossing them over each other as shown.

———— ✳ ————

10 Smooth this section of hair into a gentle curving curl.

———— ✳ ————

11 Bend back end of fine hair pin. This prevents it falling out when placed into hair.

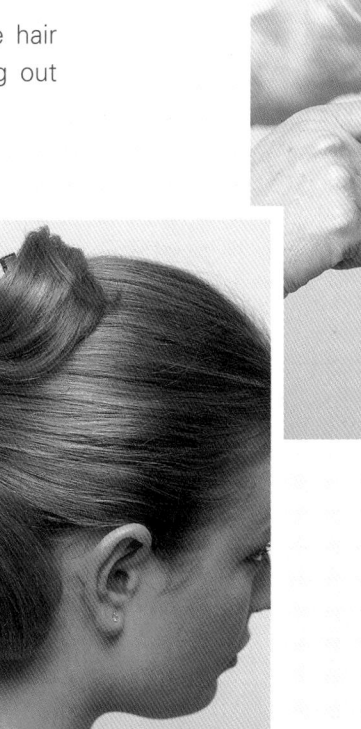

✳———————————✳

TIP

A few drops of serum worked through hair before you style will make it easier to handle and mould into shape.

✳———————————✳

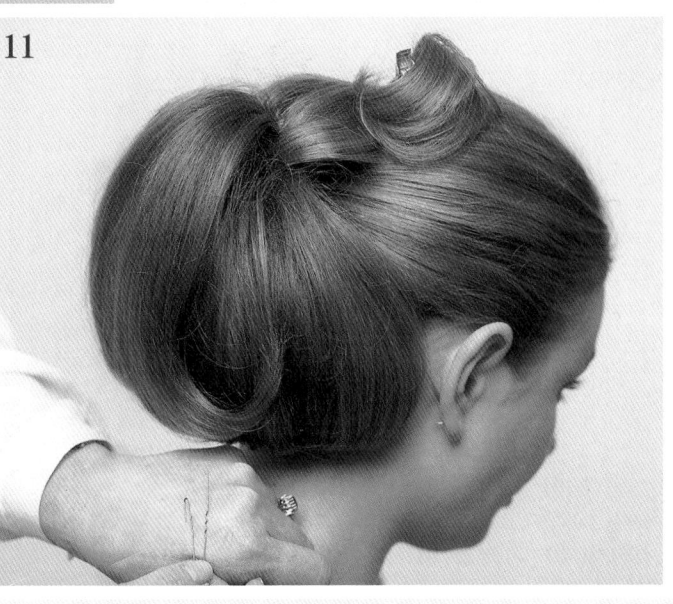

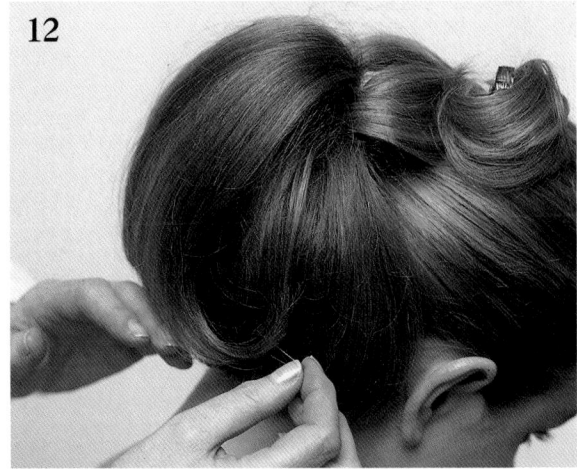

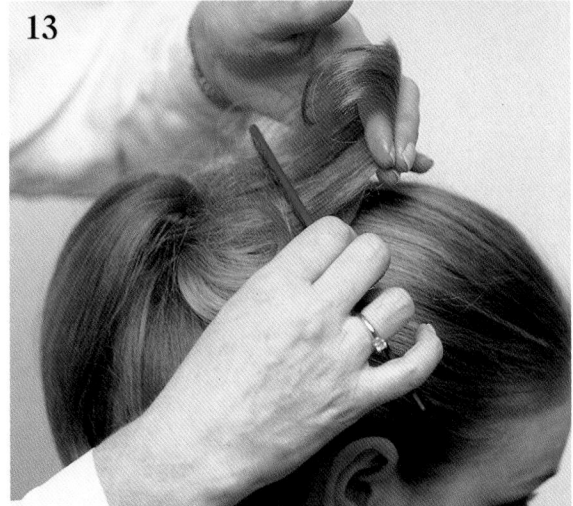

12 Use the bent pin to secure the curl.

———✳———

13 Take second reserved section of hair and backcomb.

———✳———

14 Twist into a curl.

———✳———

15 Tuck in any stray ends using a tail comb, then pin in place. Repeat with last section of reserved hair. Pin flowers in place.

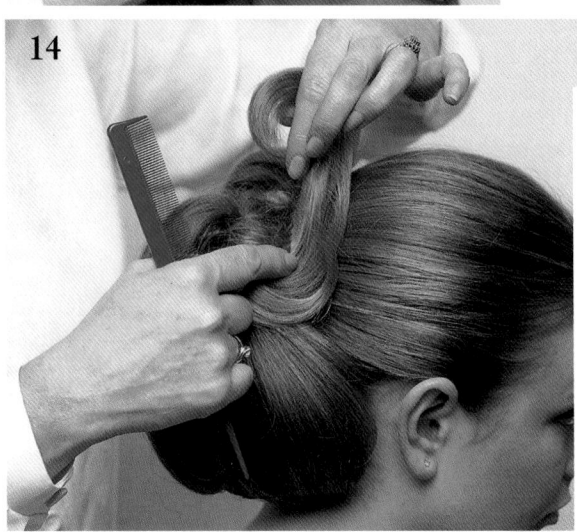

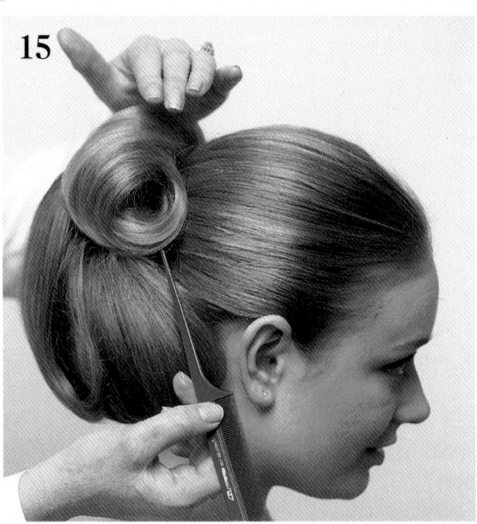

Opposite Dress: Classics Bridal Hire Collection

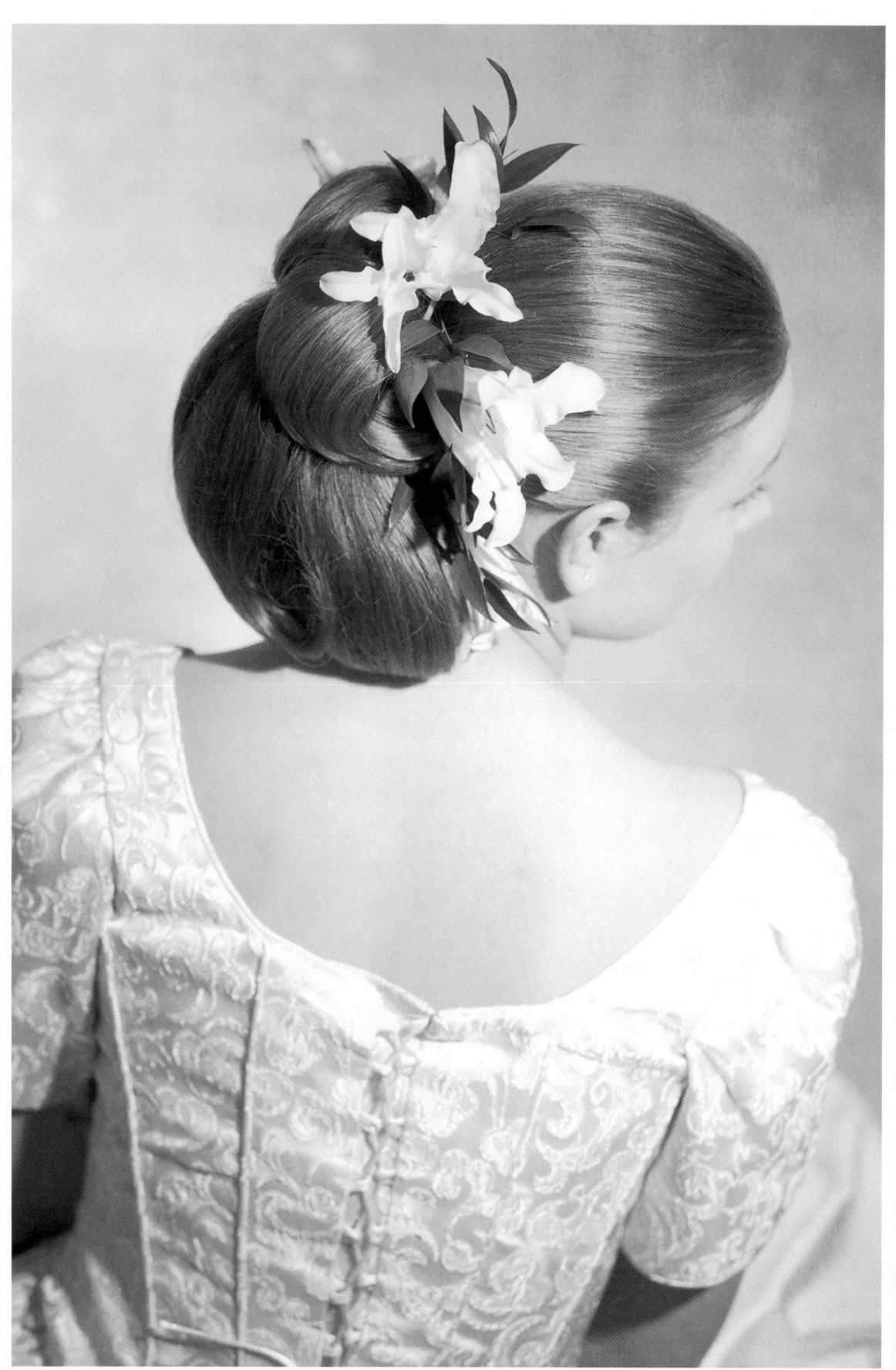

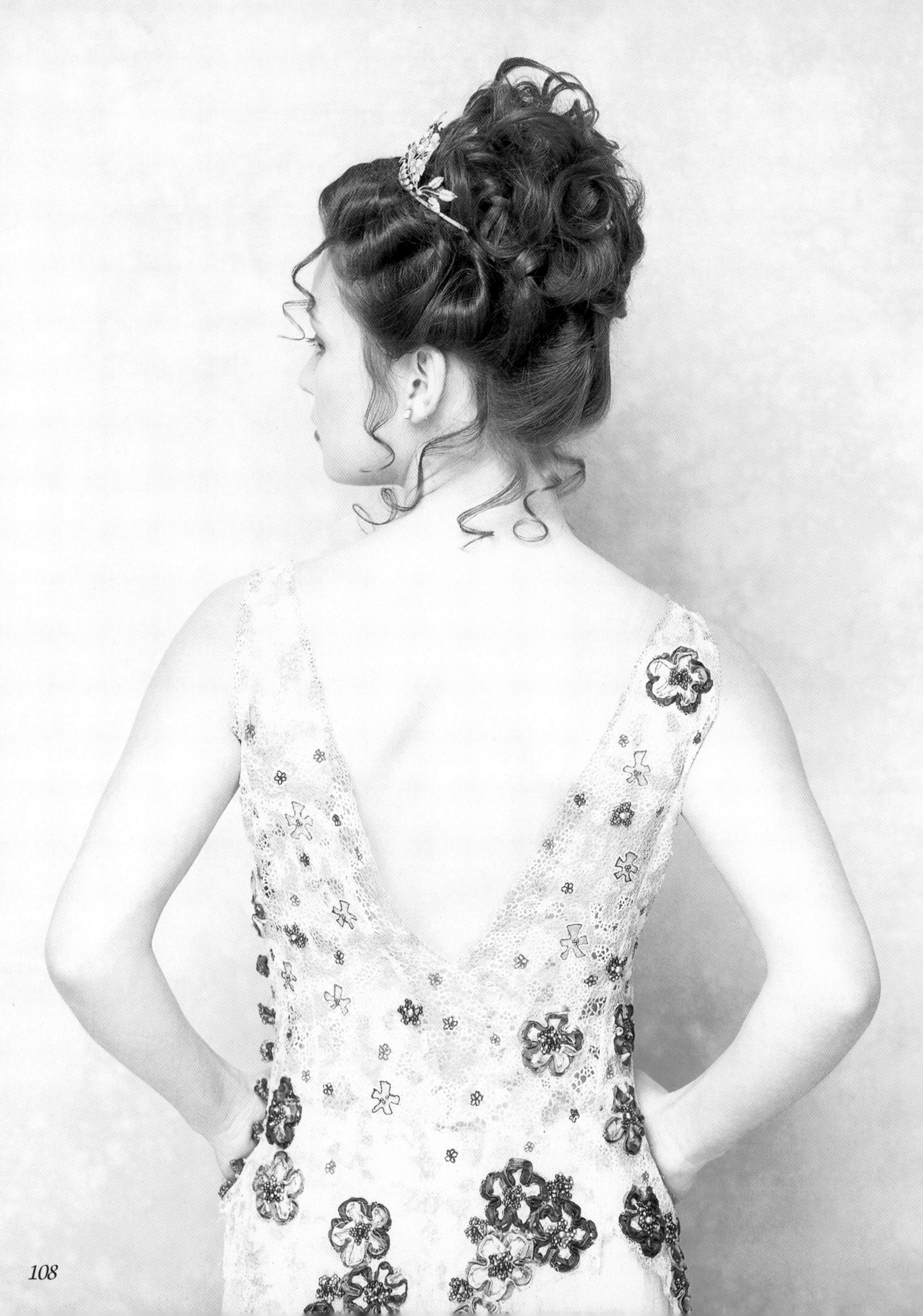

GENESSA

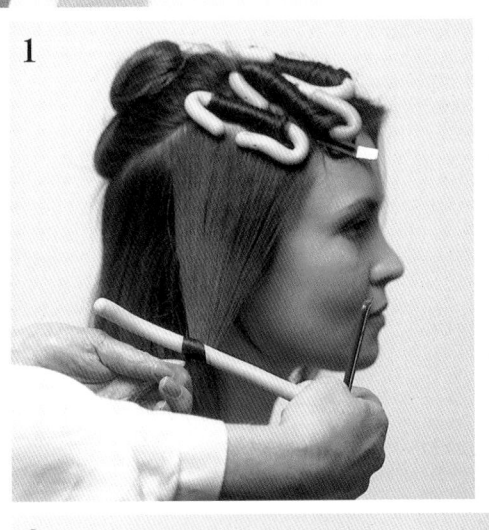

1 Section off a circle of hair on crown and clip out of the way. Set small tendrils on forehead in pin curls, then set remaining hair in hot sticks. To do this, take horizontal sections from hairline to crown. Place hot stick three inches from end of hair and wind hair over.

———— ✳ ————

2 Continue winding until you run out of hair, tucking end in so hair doesn't unravel.

———— ✳ ————

3 Wind hot stick up to scalp, tucking in any stray ends using a tail comb. Fold over each end of hot stick to secure.

———— ✳ ————

4 Shows completed side view with side tendril left free.

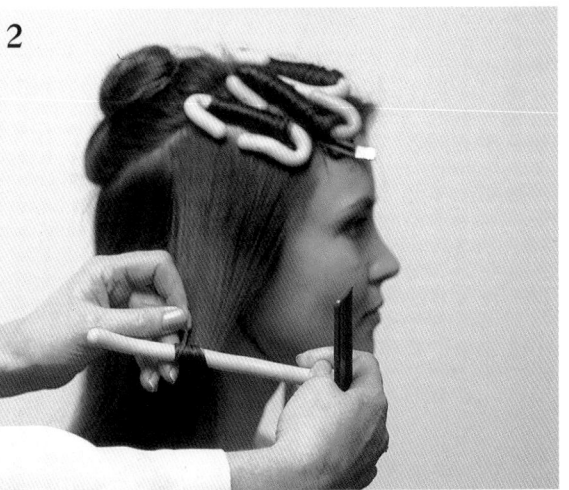

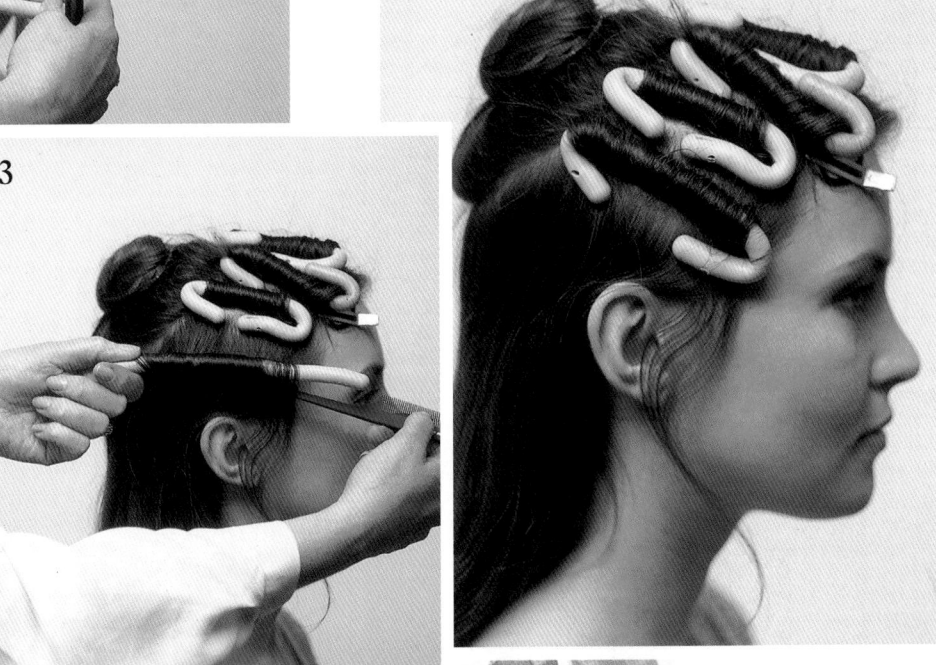

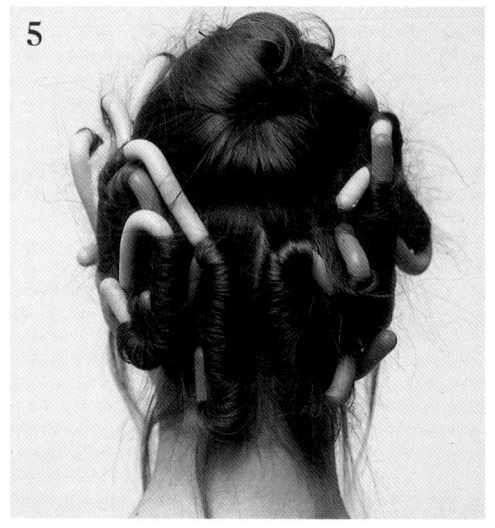

5 Continue setting hair in hot sticks in this way until all back hair is wound. Leave a few tendrils free – these will be curled later.

———— ✳ ————

6 Unclip top section of hair and set in heated rollers in the normal way.

———— ✳ ————

7 Tong side and back tendrils using a medium barrel tong.

———— ✳ ————

8 Remove hot sticks by first straightening folded over ends and unwinding a little way.

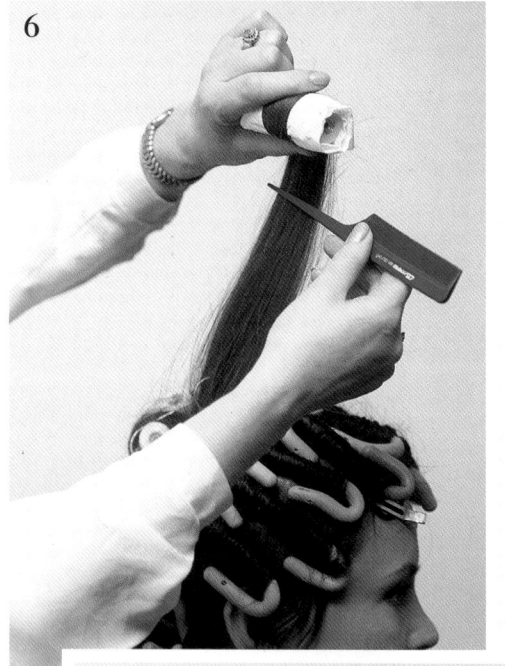

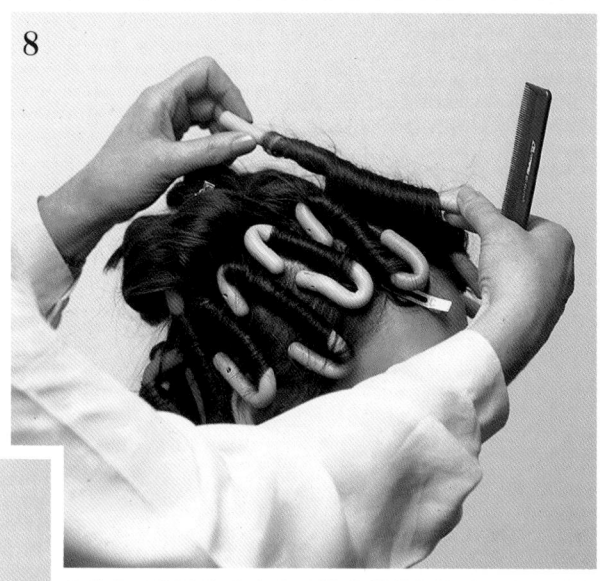

✳ ———————————— ✳

TIP

Take care not to buckle ends of hair when using hot sticks or heated rollers.

✳ ———————————— ✳

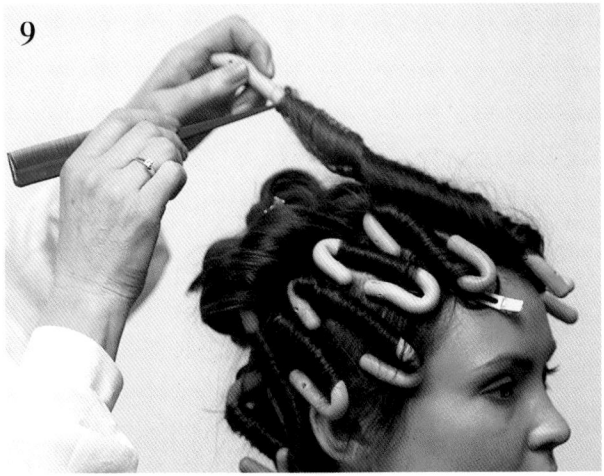

9 Gently loosen the hot stick and start to remove, allowing coil of hair to stay in place. Encourage coil to stay in place using the end of a tail comb.

———— ❋ ————

10 Carefully pull out hot stick.

———— ❋ ————

11 Tie end of hair into a loose knot.

———— ❋ ————

12 Grip curl in place at base of knot.

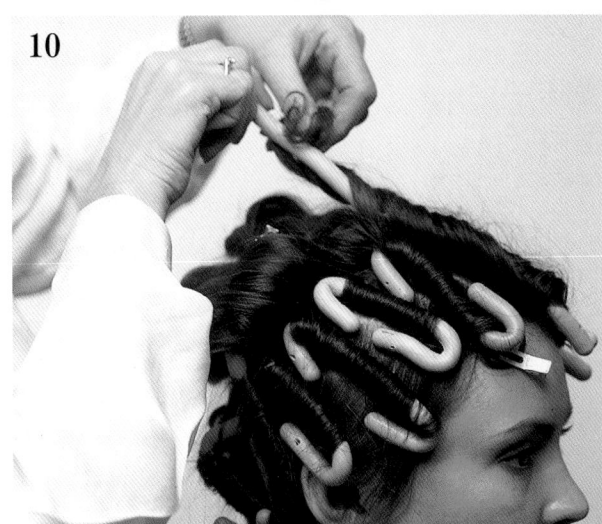

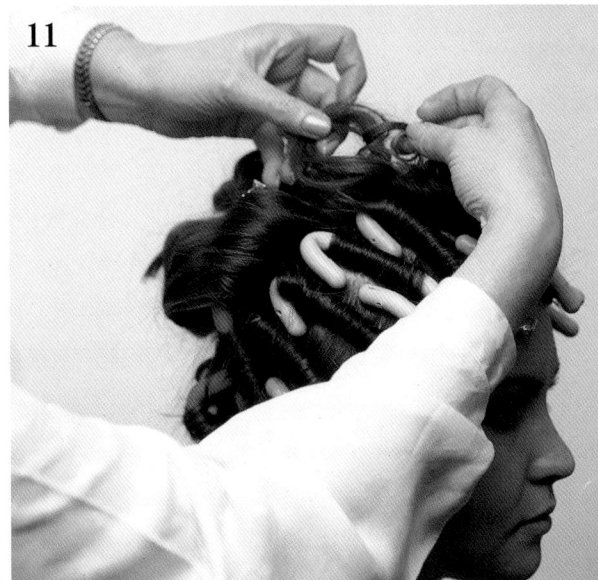

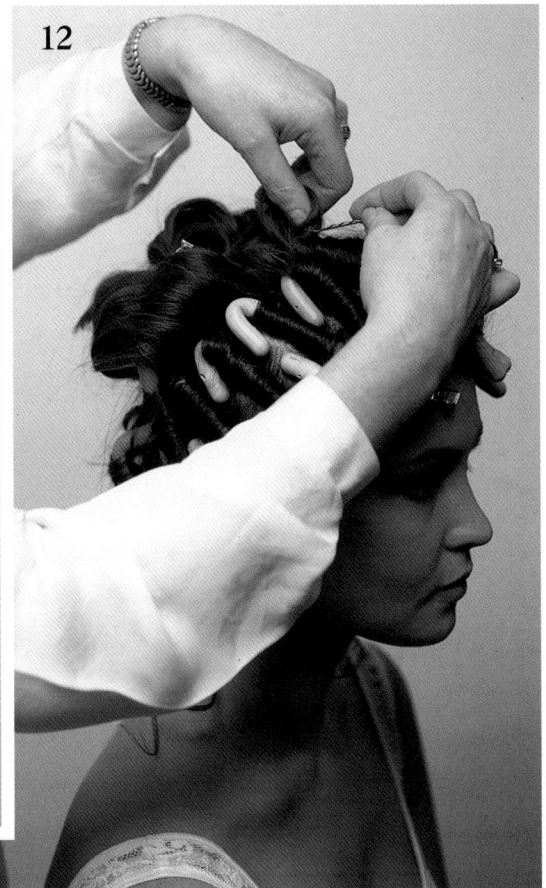

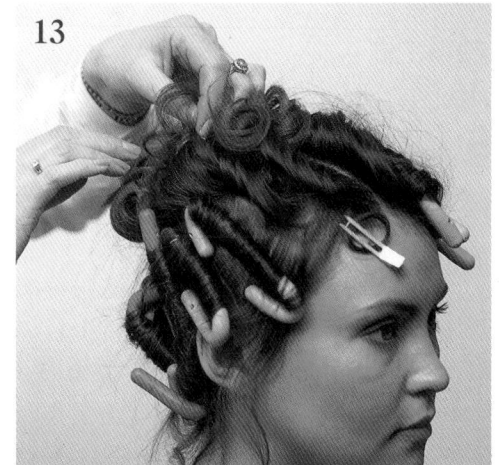
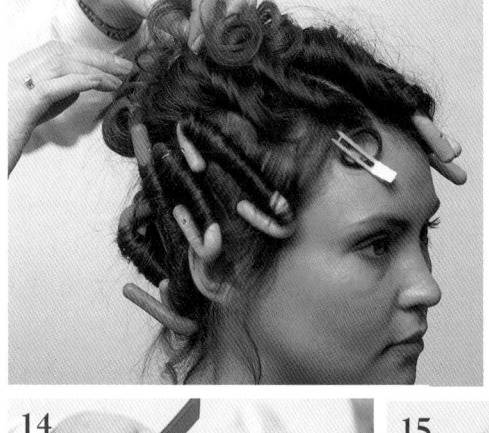

13 Remove heated rollers and loop hair into curls.

———— ✳ ————

14 Continue working in same way until all curls are formed and pinned.

———— ✳ ————

15 Tidy any stray ends using a tail comb.

———— ✳ ————

16 Release front pin curls and secure hair at back with pins.

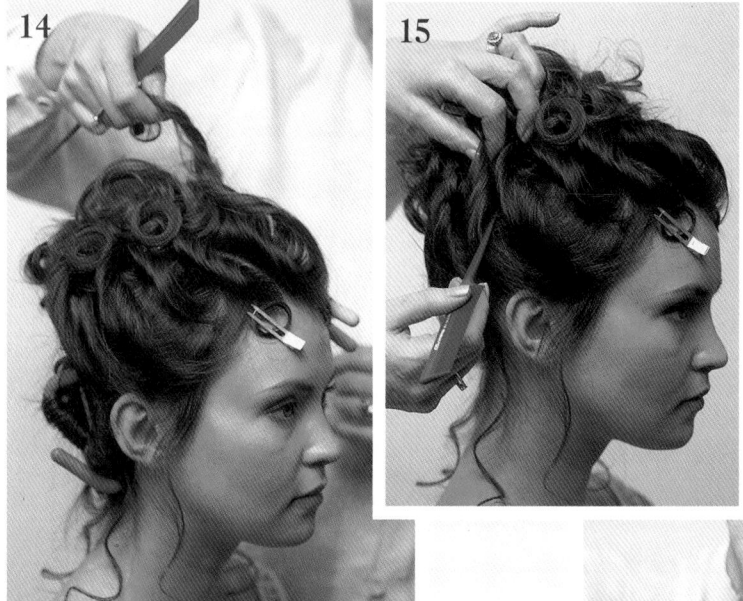

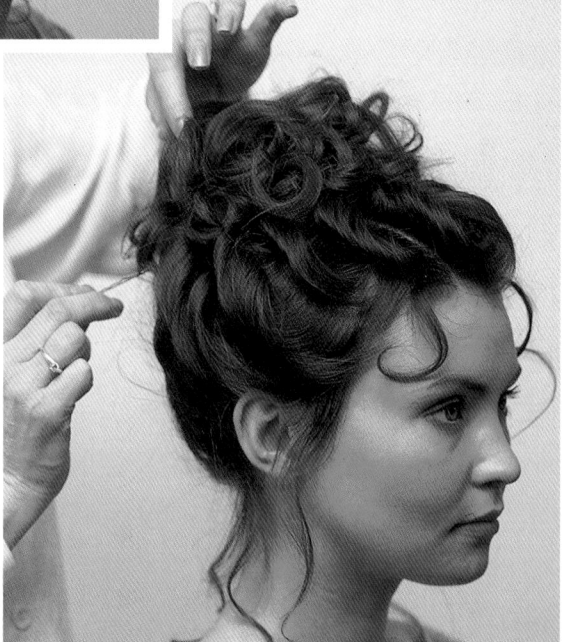

Opposite Dress and head-dress: Kesté by Myring Kesterton

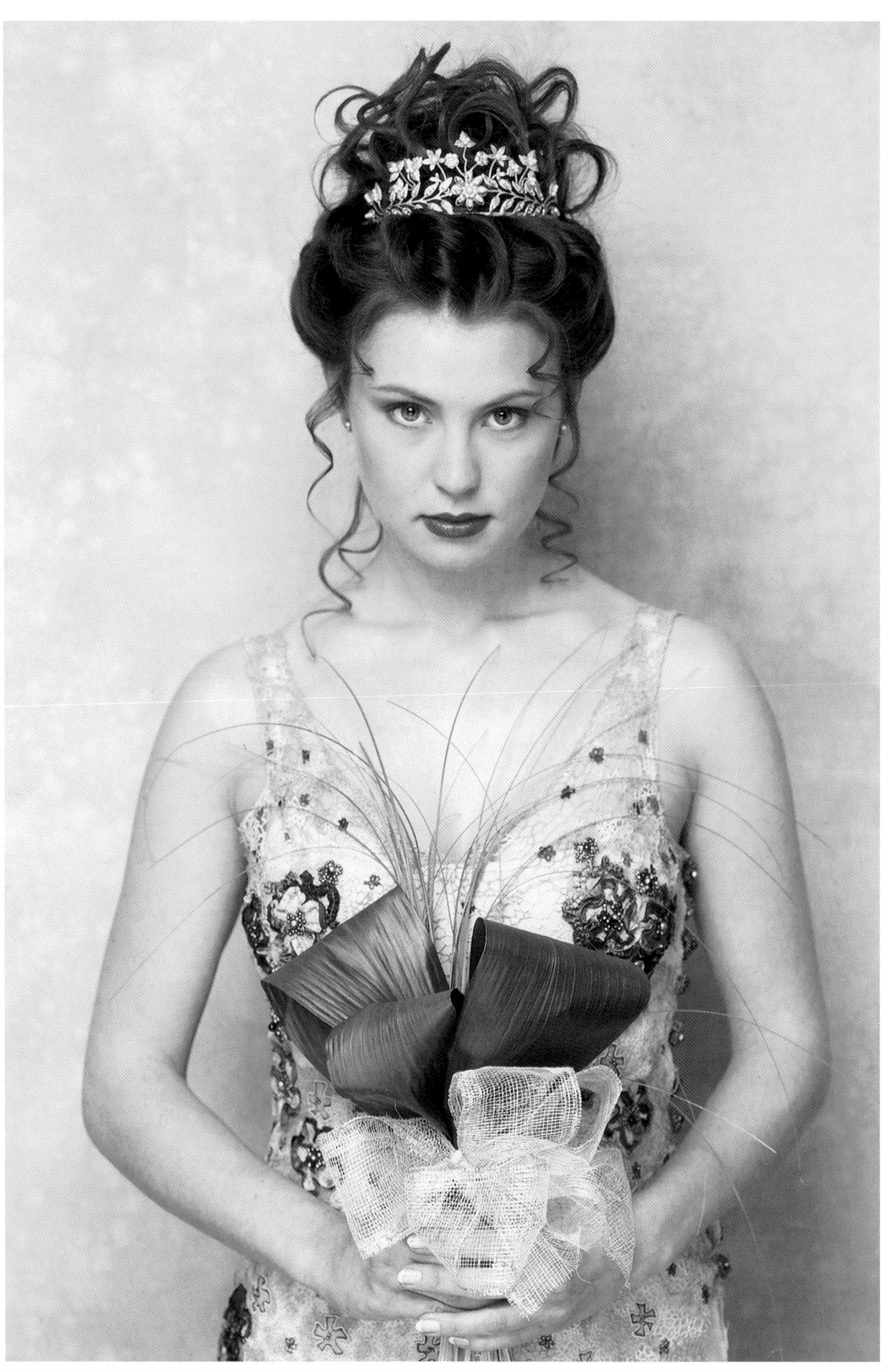

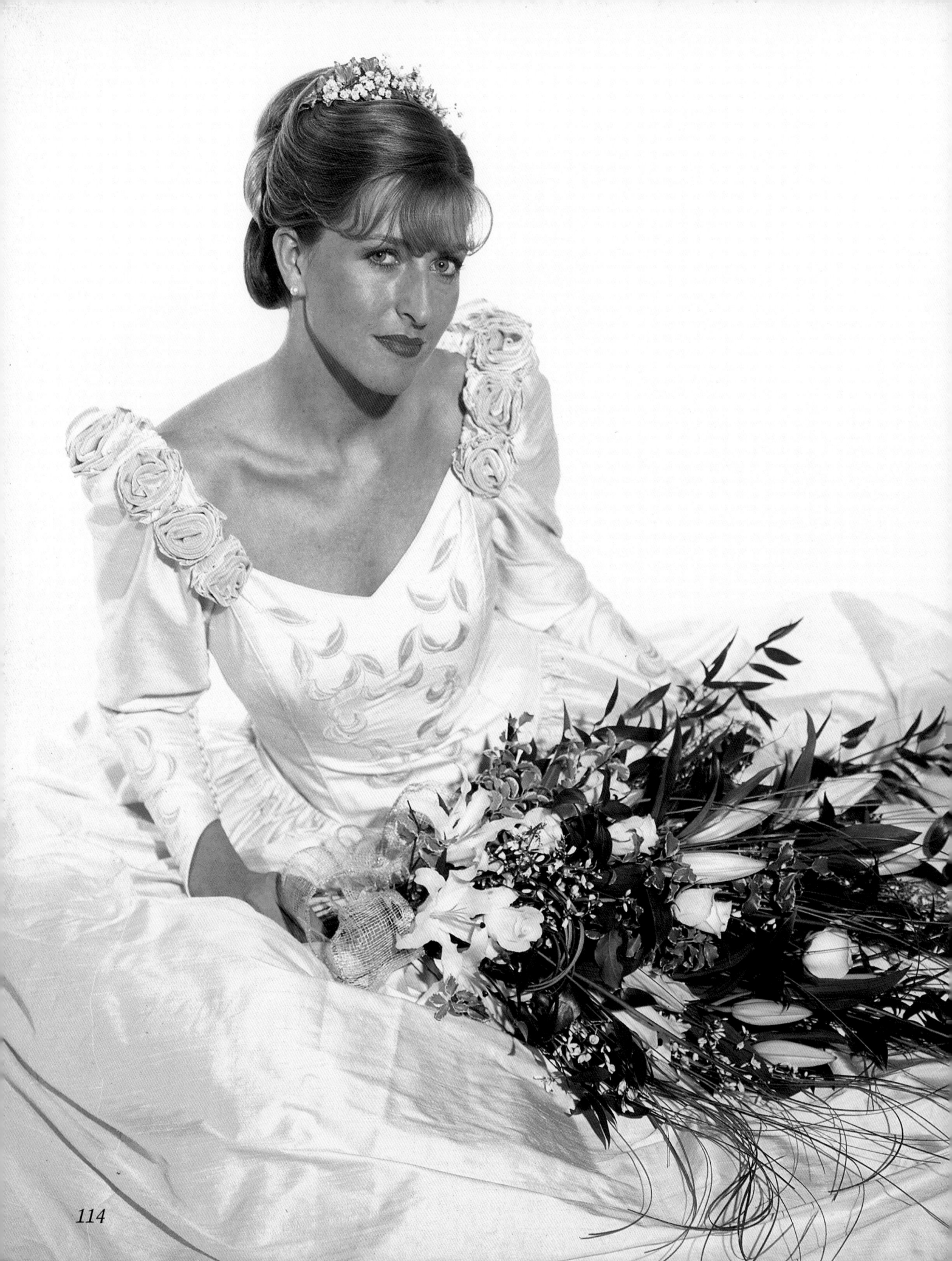

IVY

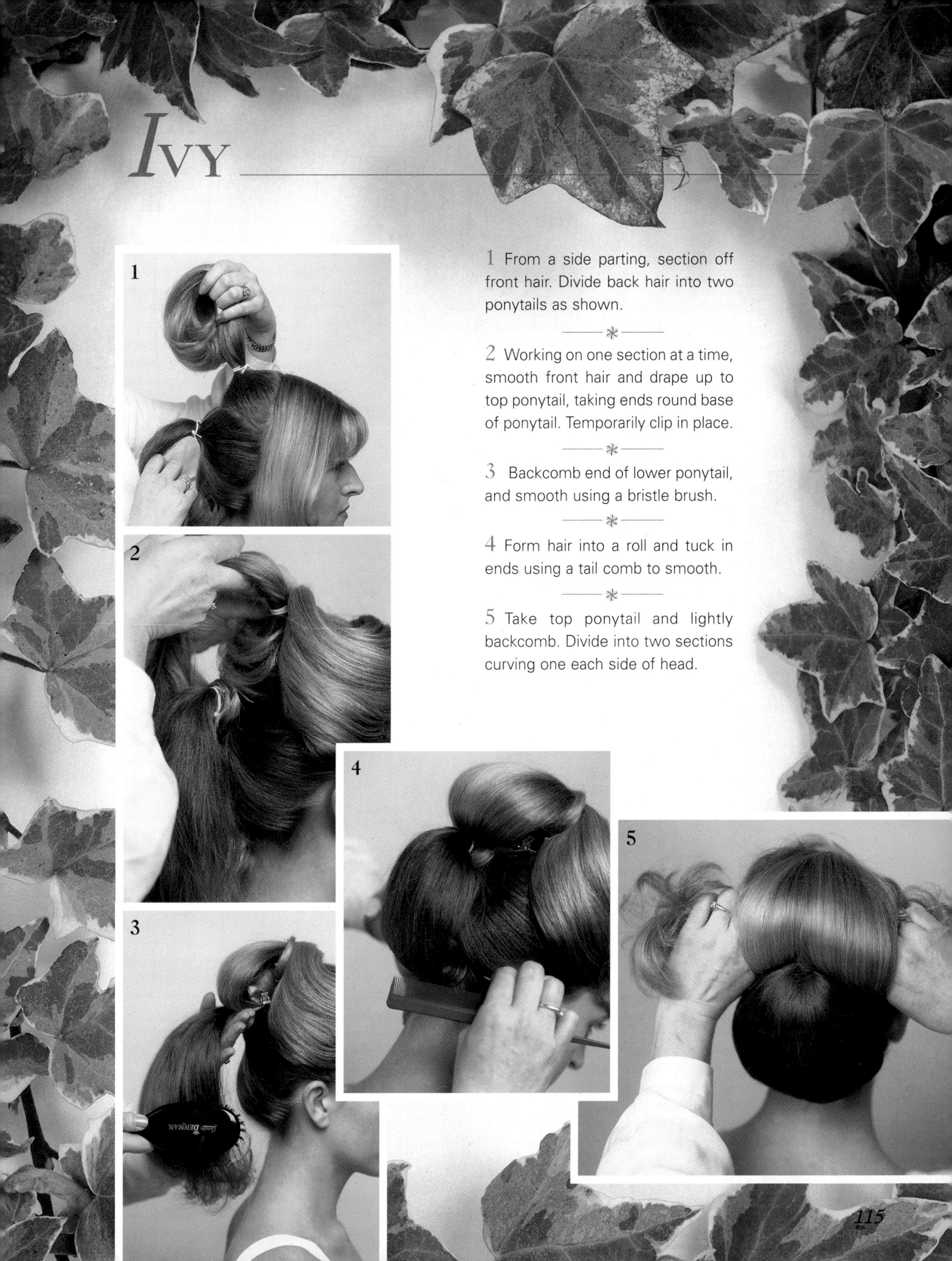

1 From a side parting, section off front hair. Divide back hair into two ponytails as shown.

———— ✳ ————

2 Working on one section at a time, smooth front hair and drape up to top ponytail, taking ends round base of ponytail. Temporarily clip in place.

———— ✳ ————

3 Backcomb end of lower ponytail, and smooth using a bristle brush.

———— ✳ ————

4 Form hair into a roll and tuck in ends using a tail comb to smooth.

———— ✳ ————

5 Take top ponytail and lightly backcomb. Divide into two sections curving one each side of head.

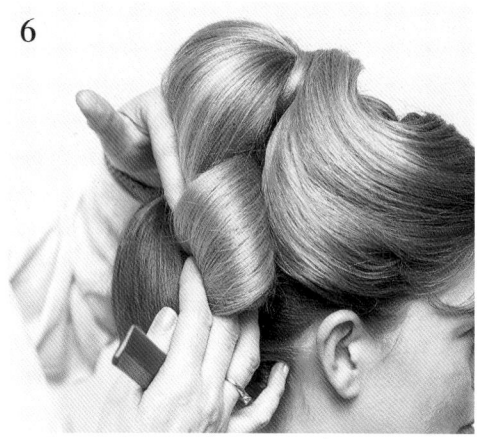

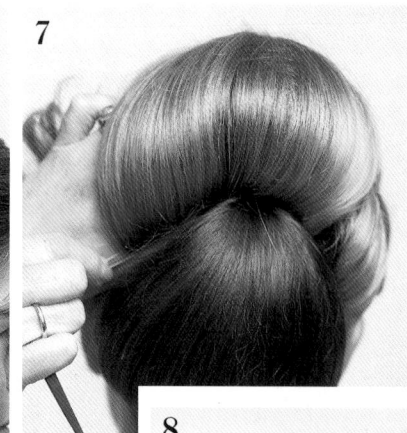

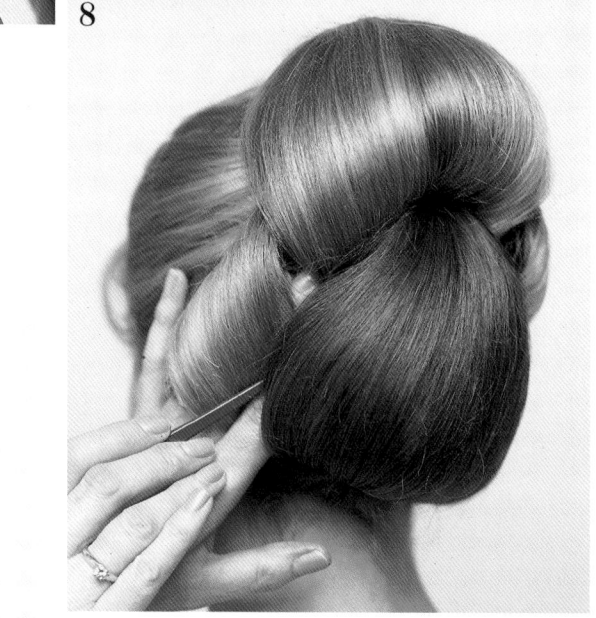

6 Lightly twist ends of one of these sections round fingers, using a tail comb to tuck in ends, then secure with grips and pins.

———— ✳ ————

7 Repeat for other side, first curving the section of hair ...

———— ✳ ————

8 ... then coiling, tucking ends in and pinning into place.

———— ✳ ————

9 Shows completed back view.

———— ✳ ————

10 Position floral headband and secure with grips.

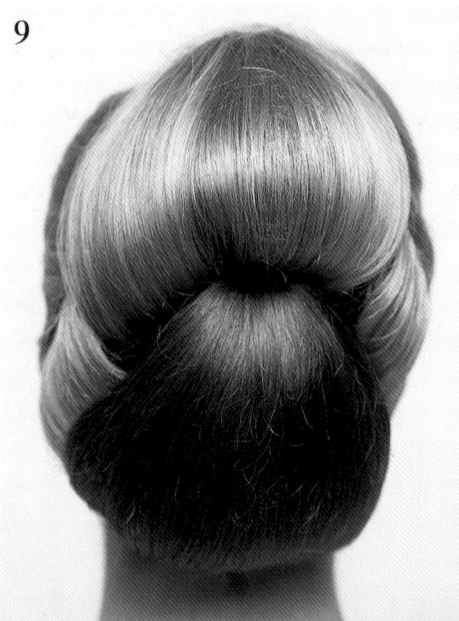

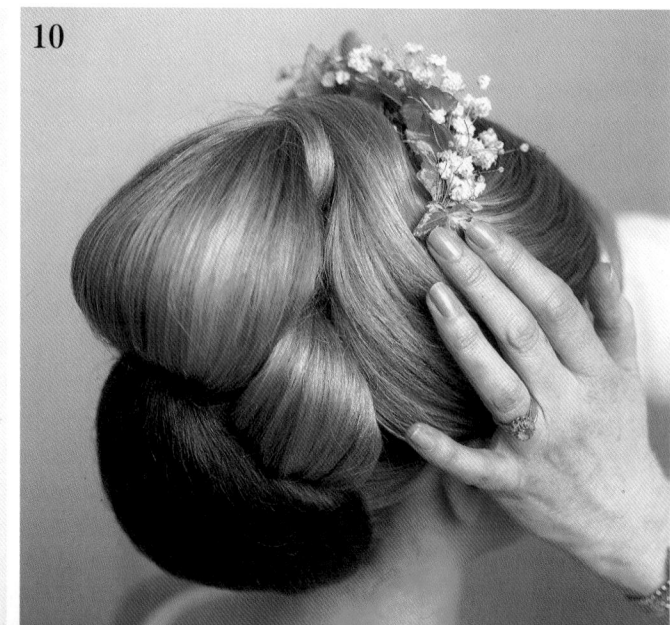

Seasonal & themed wedding styles

SPRING

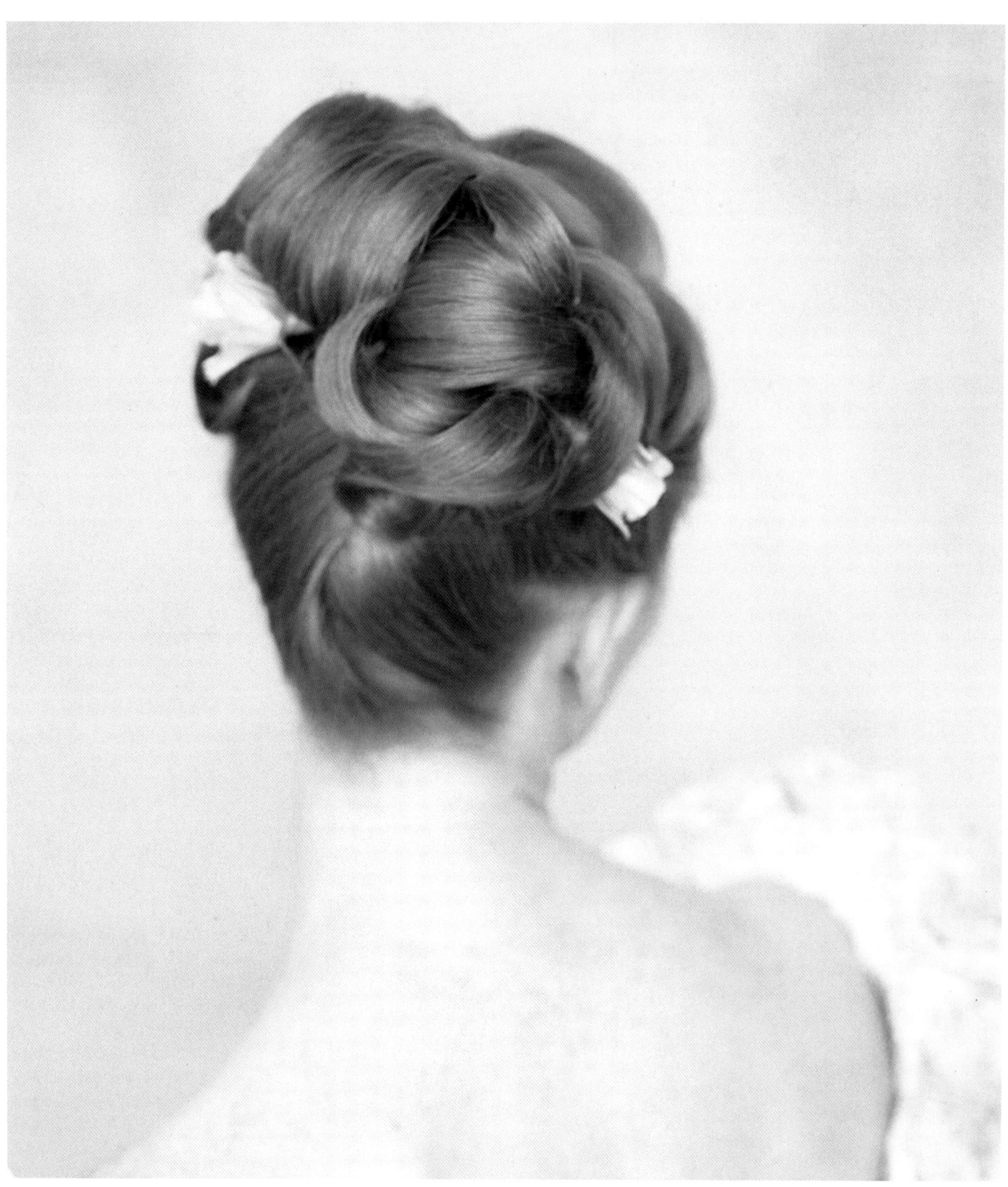

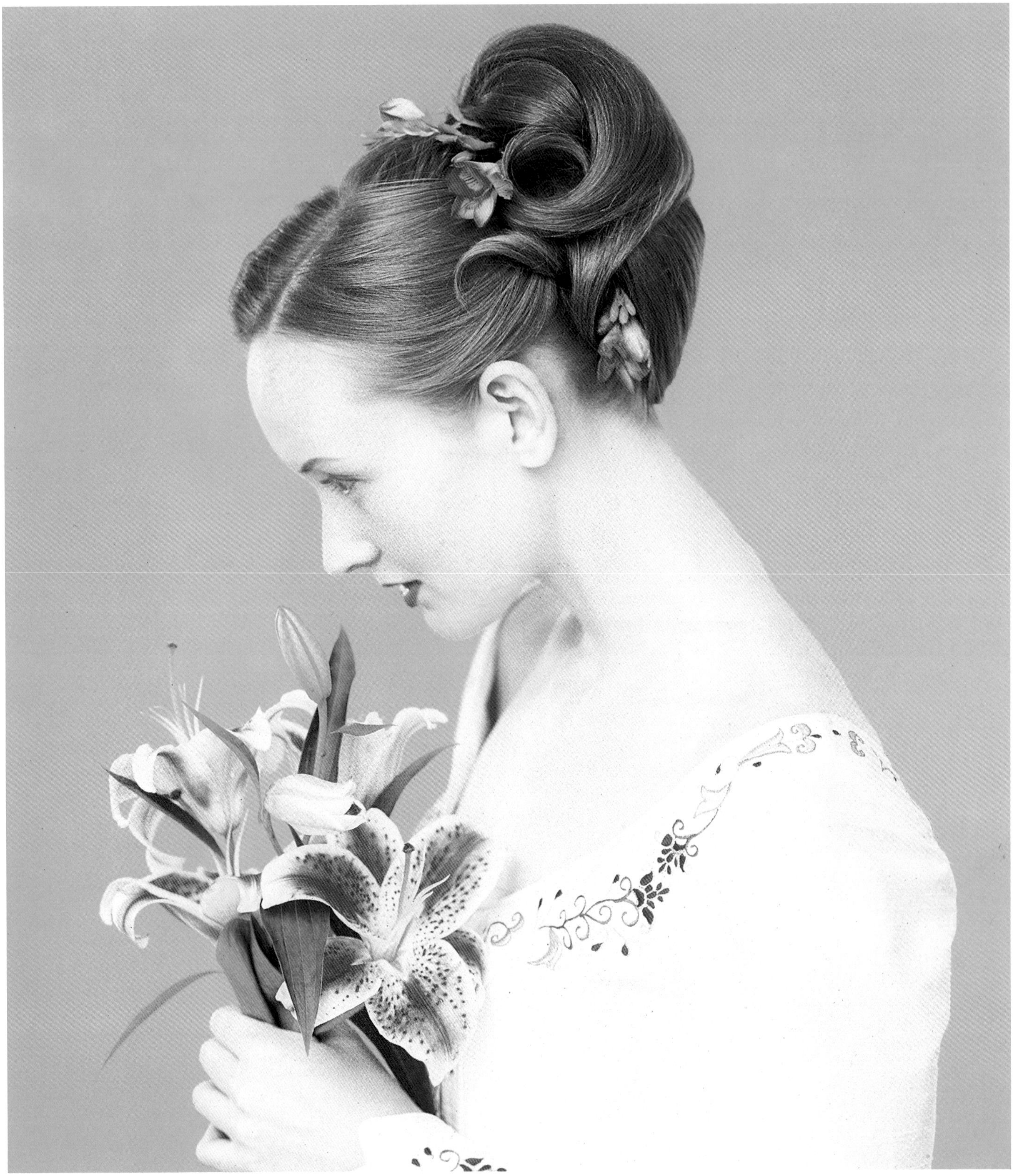

SUMMER

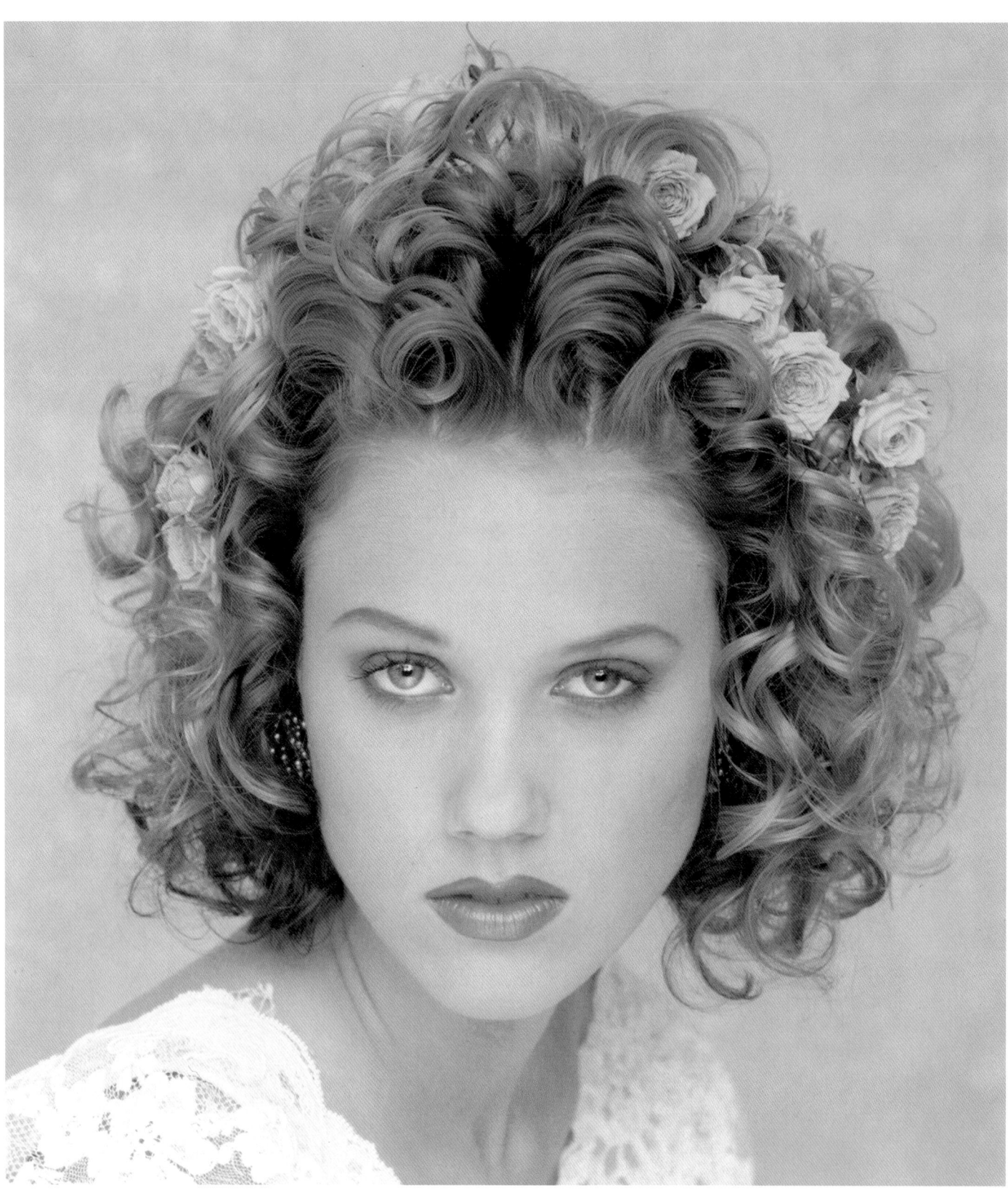

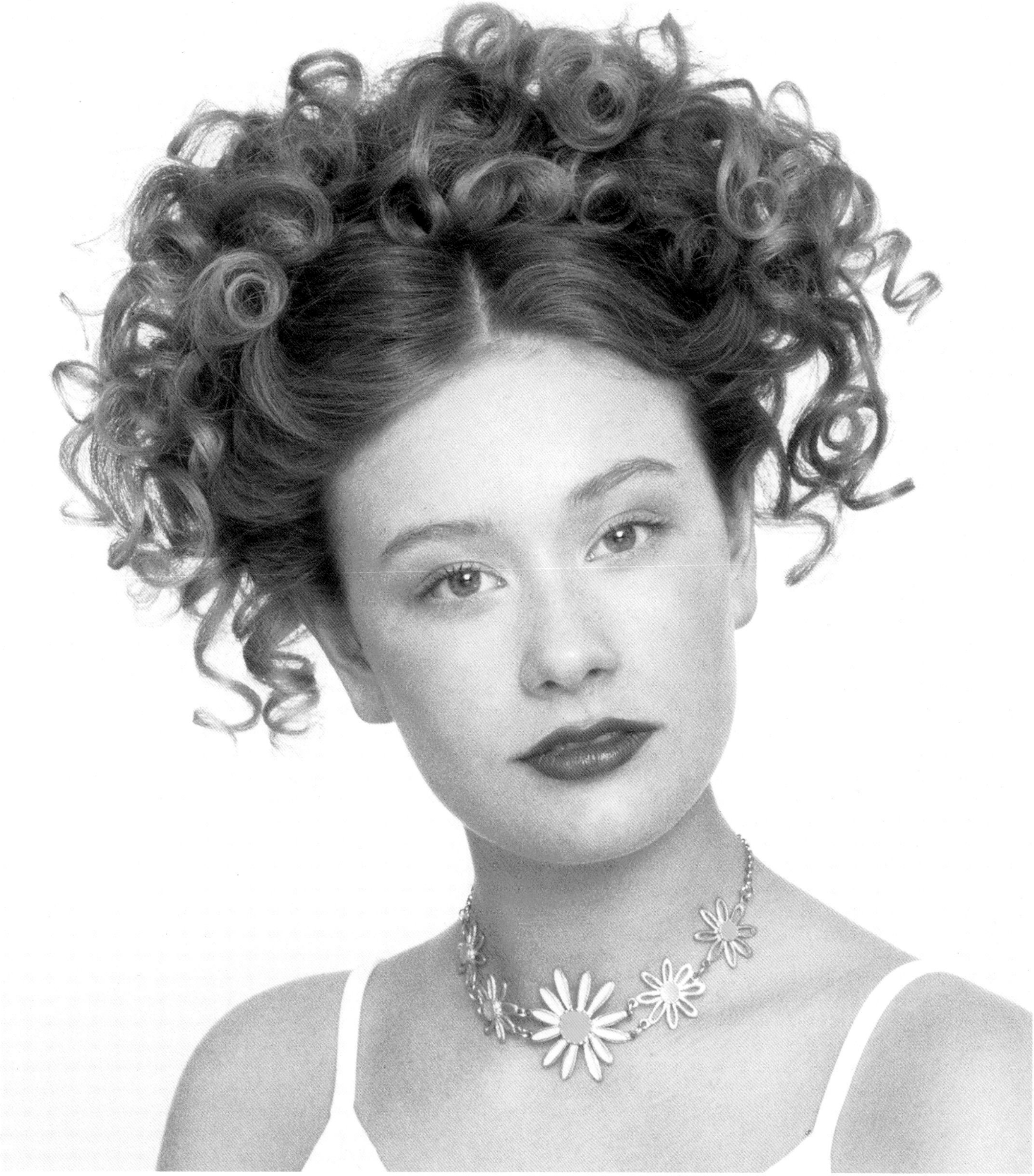

AUTUMN

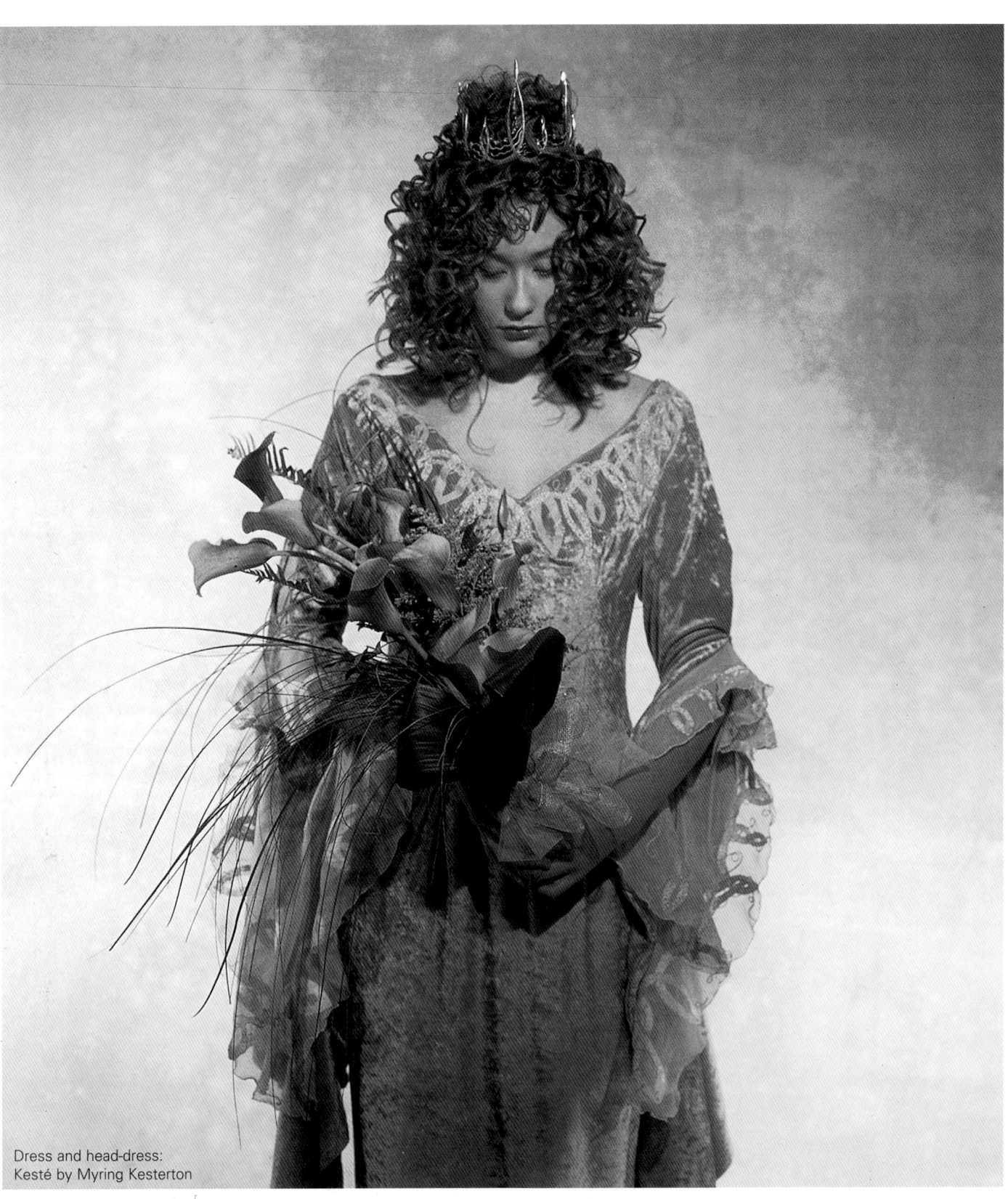

Dress and head-dress:
Kesté by Myring Kesterton

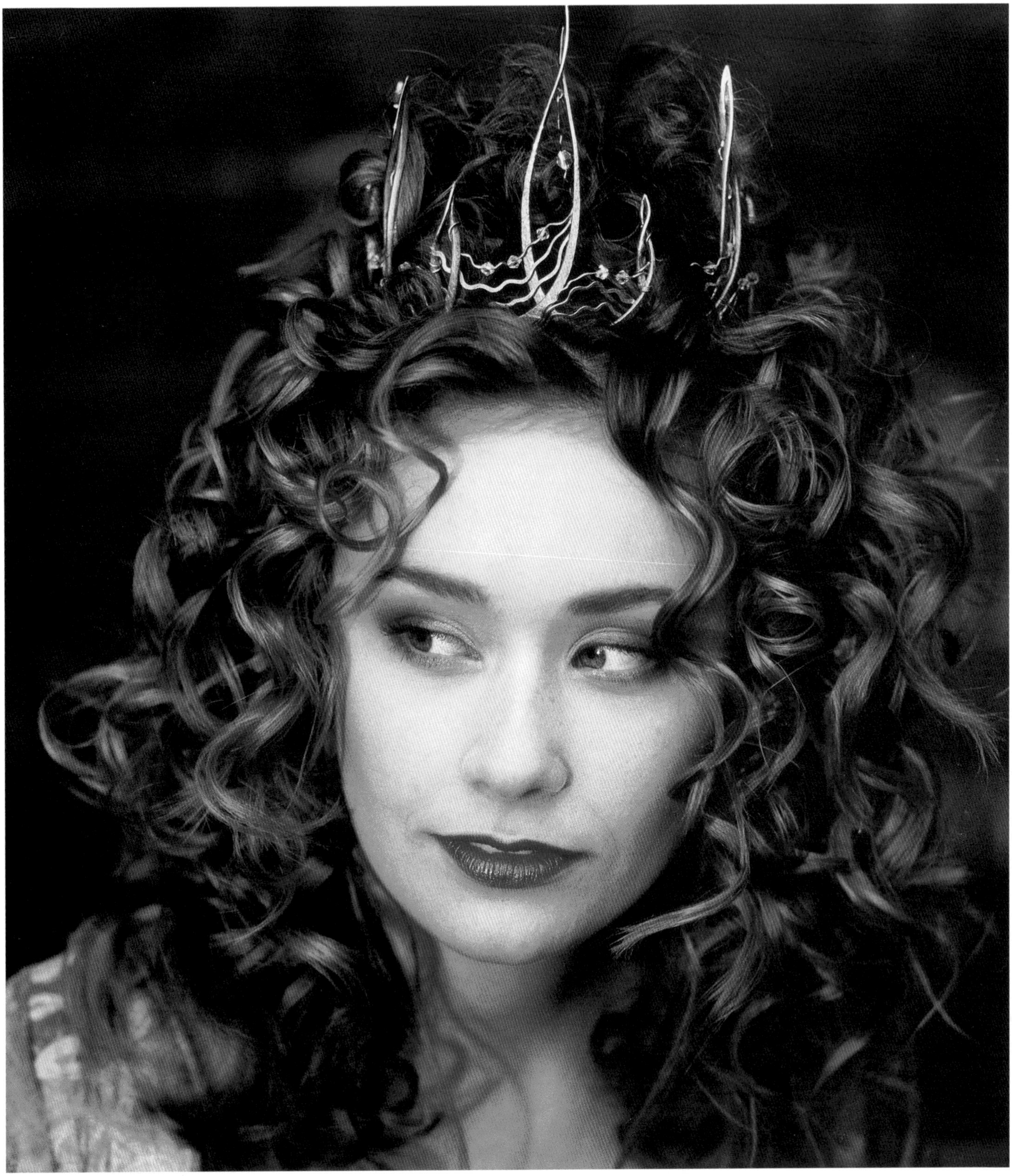

WINTER

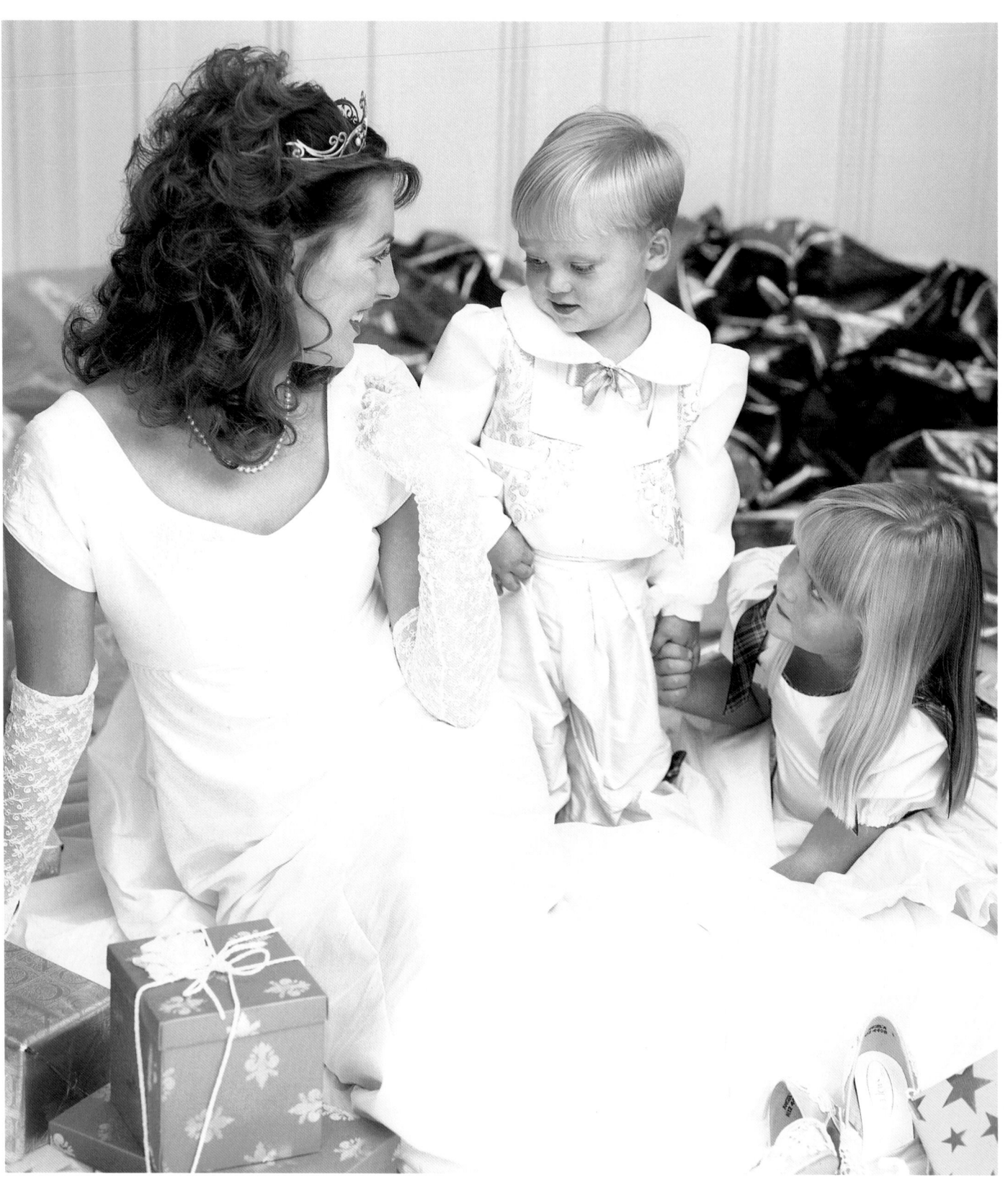

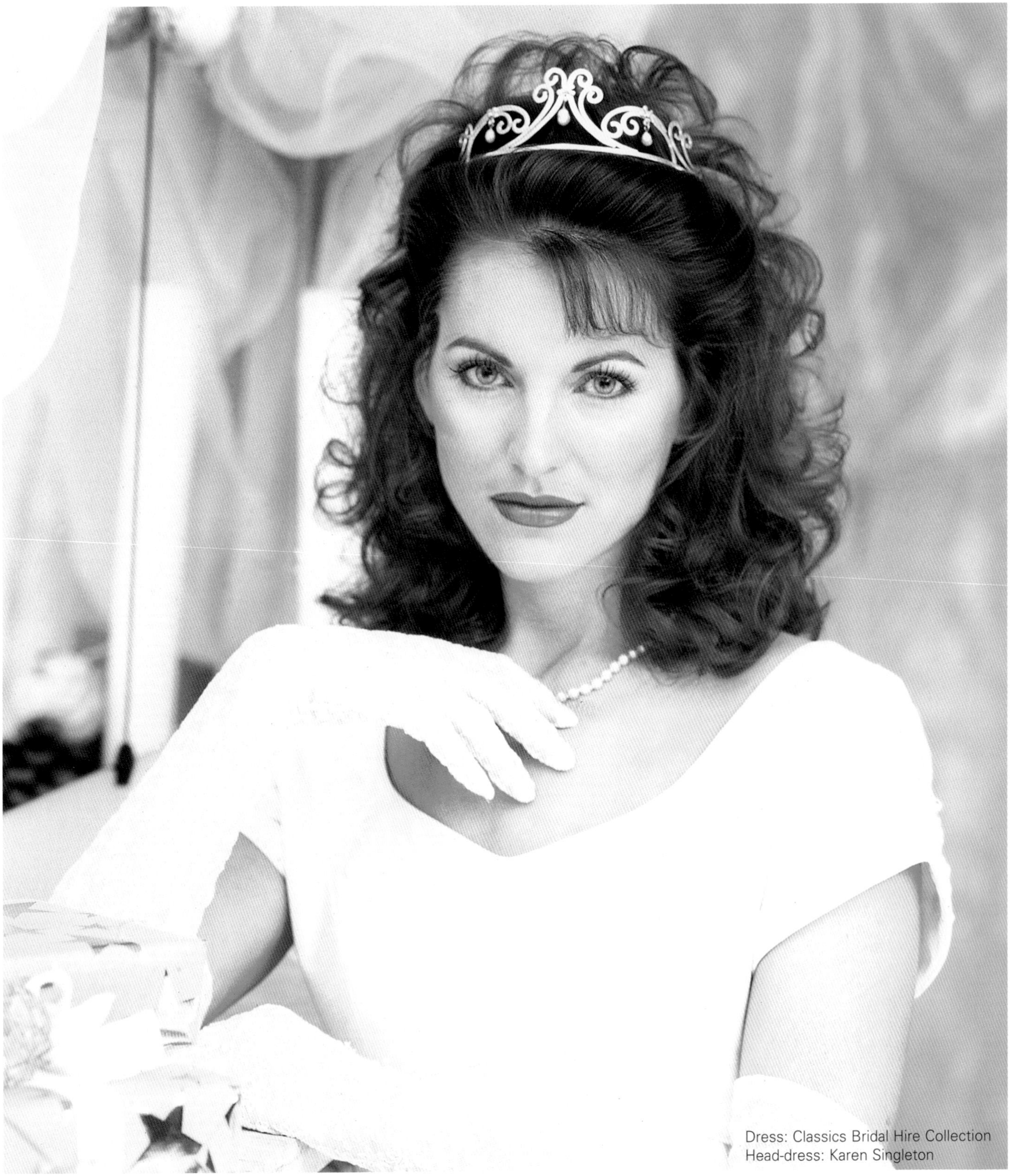

Dress: Classics Bridal Hire Collection
Head-dress: Karen Singleton

Medieval

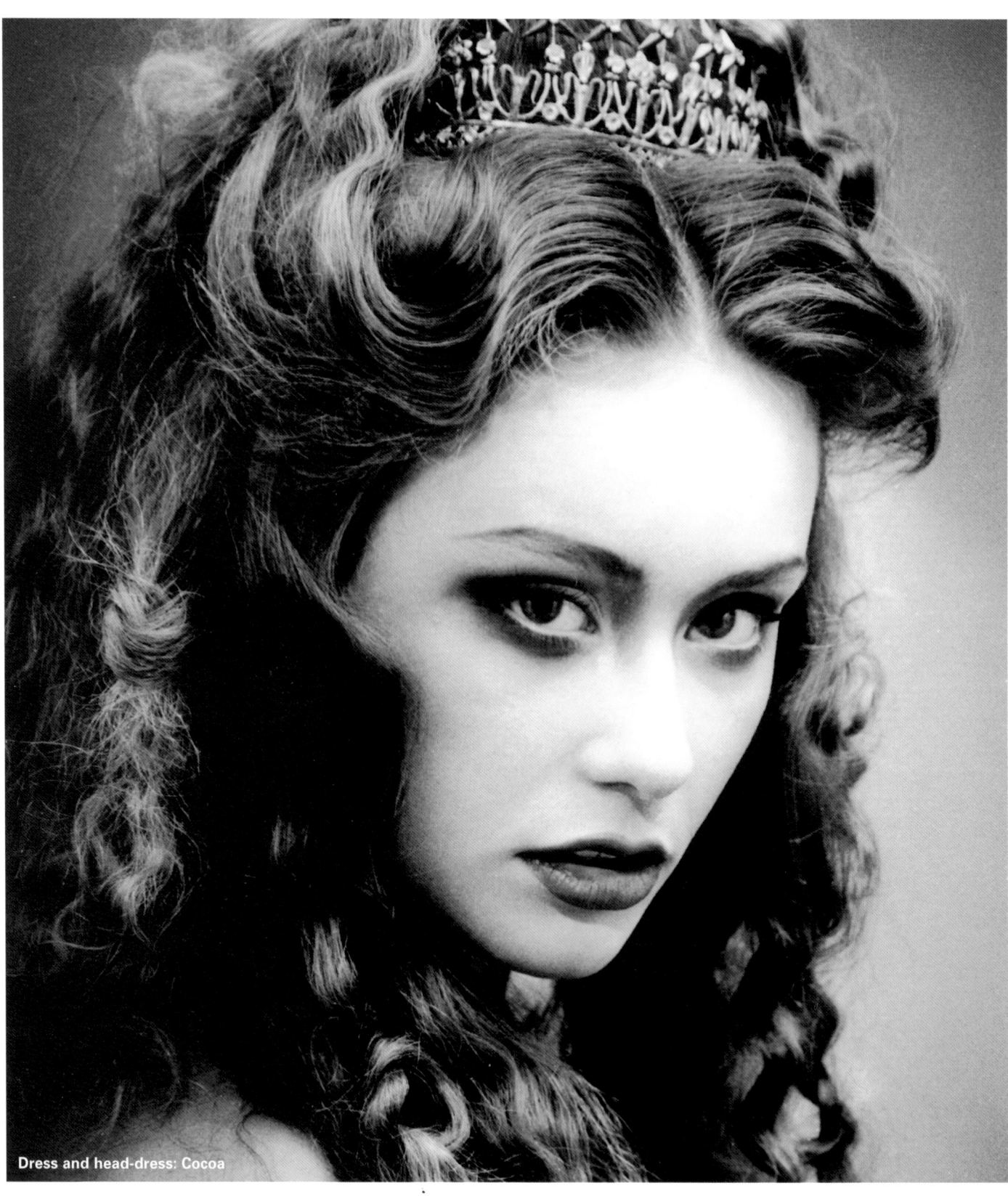

Dress and head-dress: Cocoa

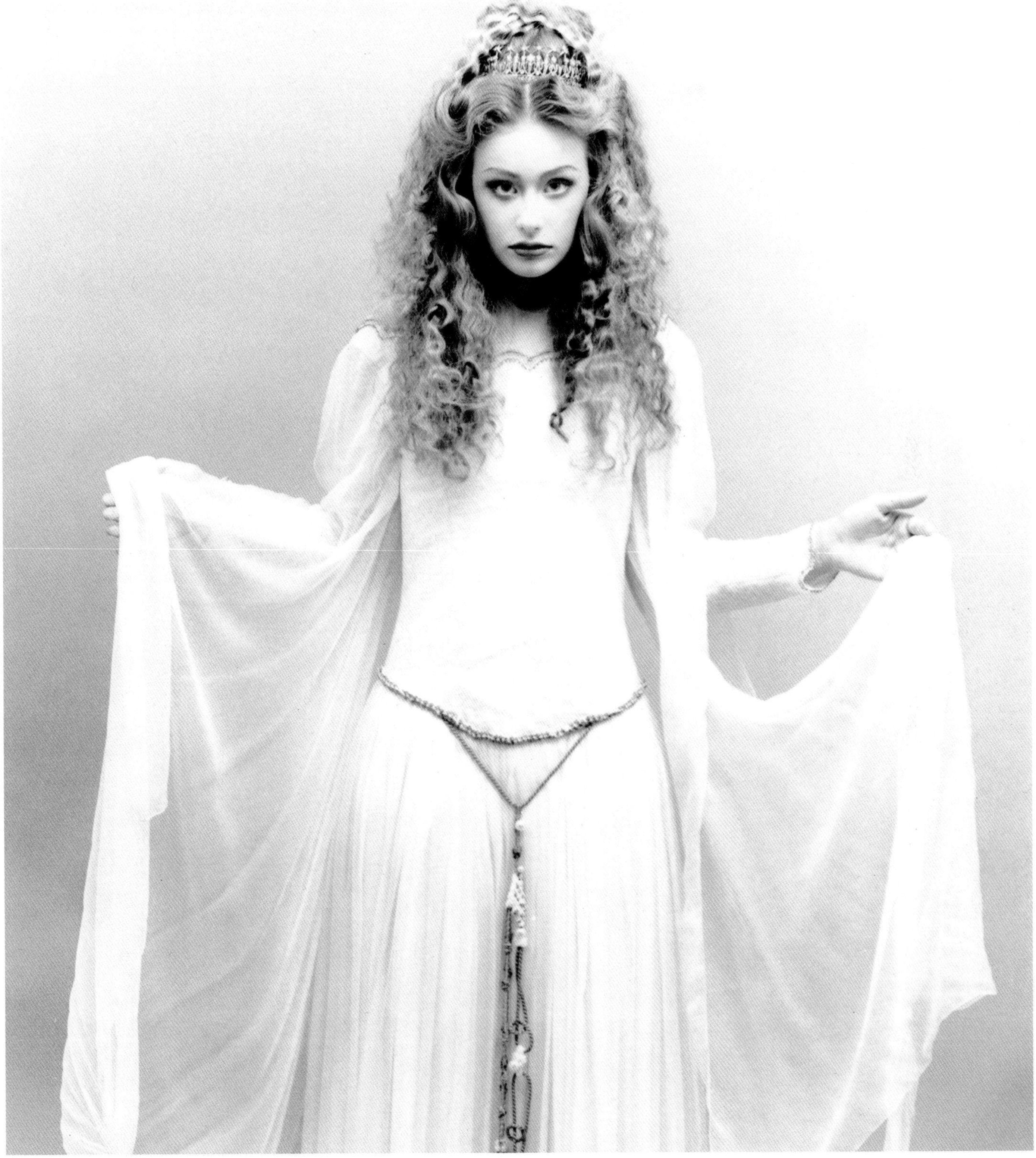

CLASSICAL

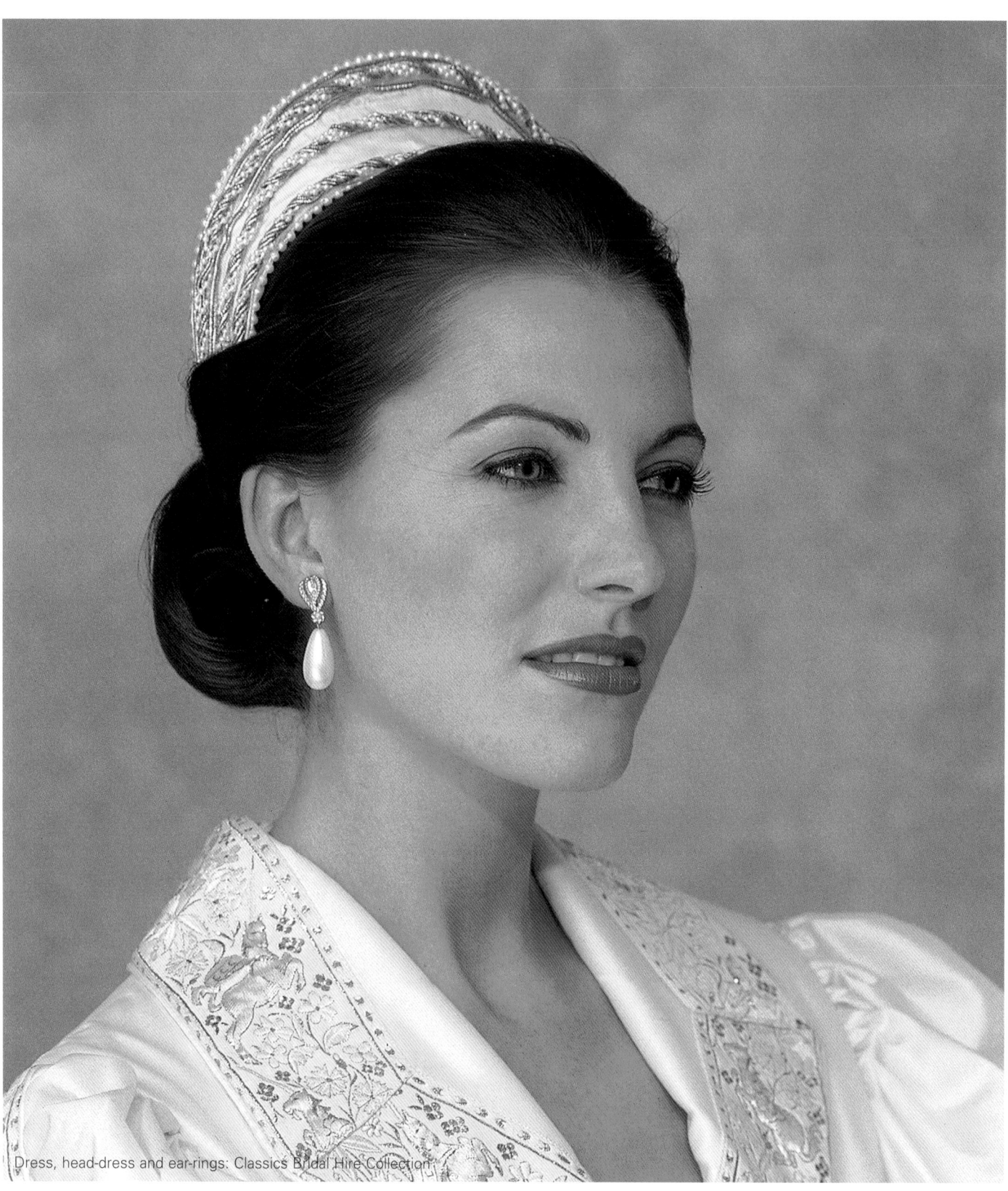

Dress, head-dress and ear-rings: Classics Bridal Hire Collection

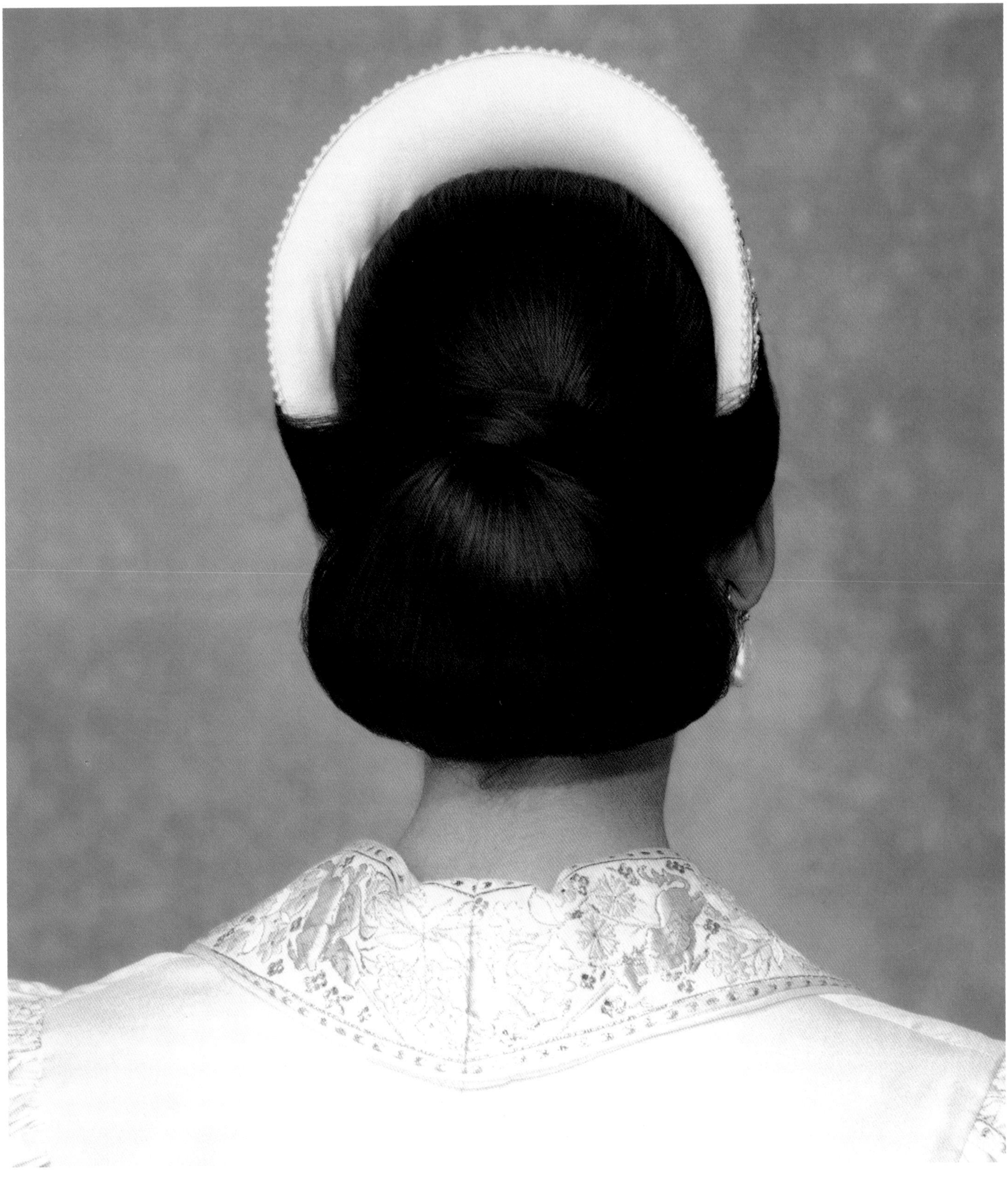

TRADITIONAL

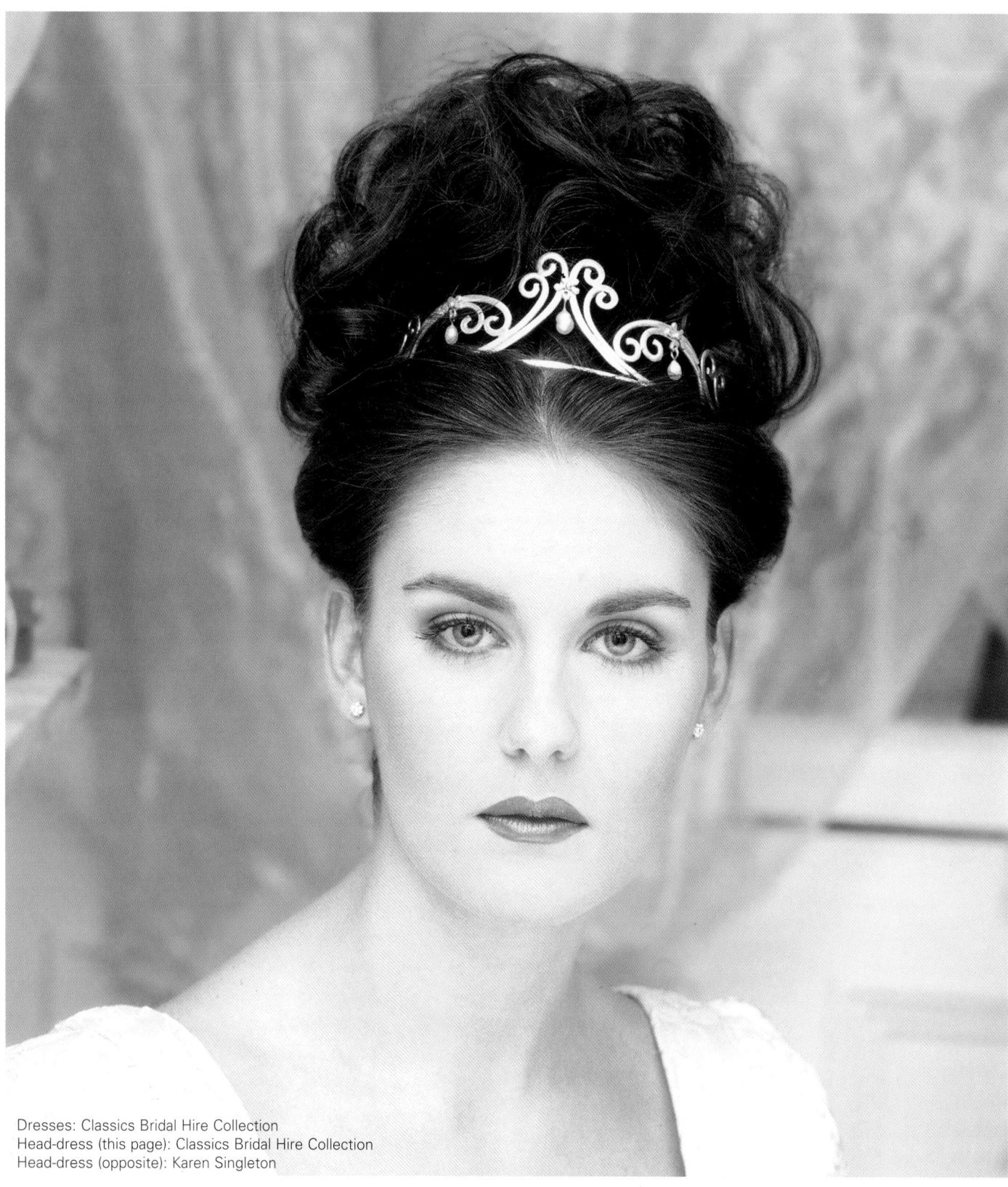

Dresses: Classics Bridal Hire Collection
Head-dress (this page): Classics Bridal Hire Collection
Head-dress (opposite): Karen Singleton

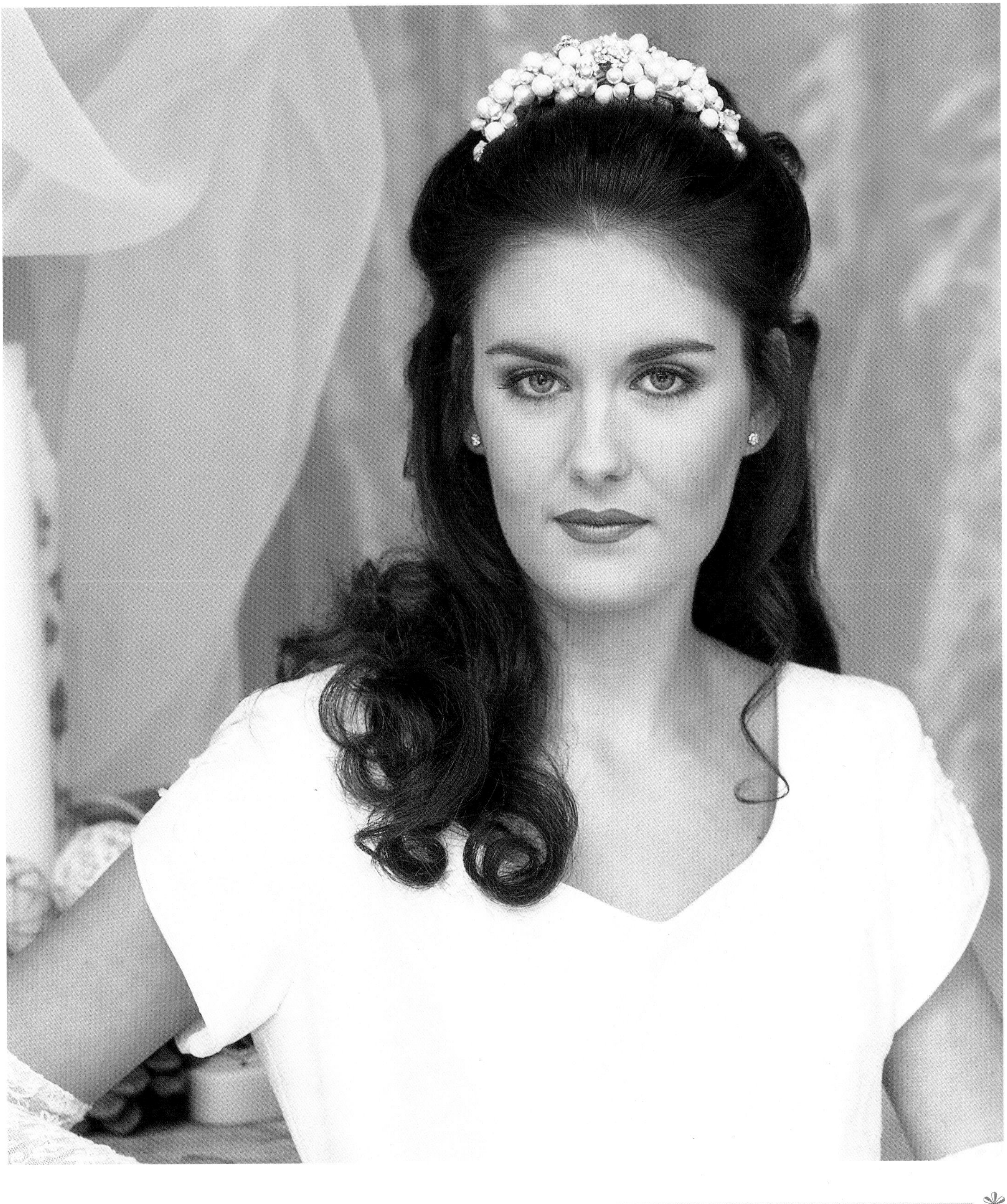

MODERN

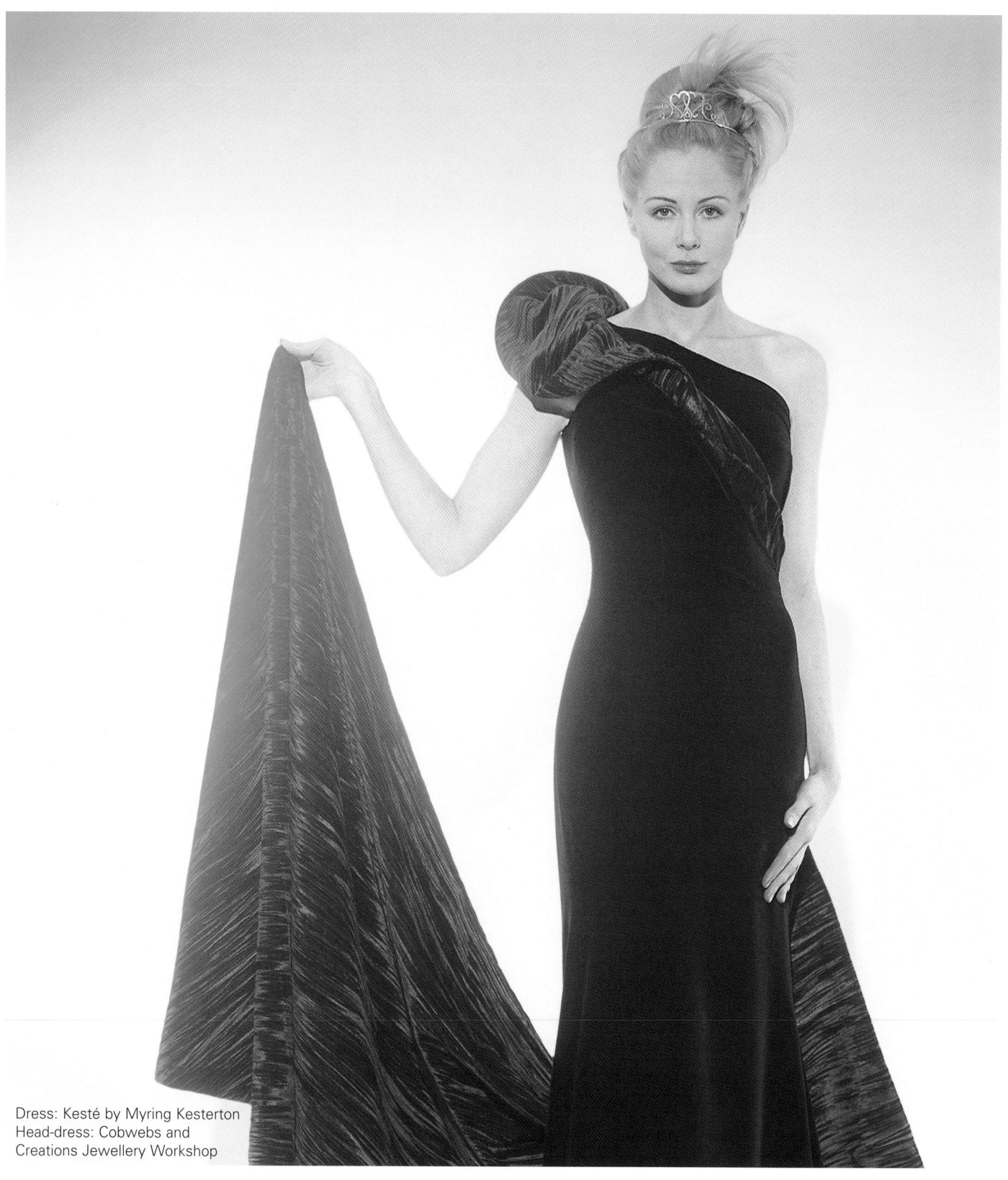

Dress: Kesté by Myring Kesterton
Head-dress: Cobwebs and
Creations Jewellery Workshop

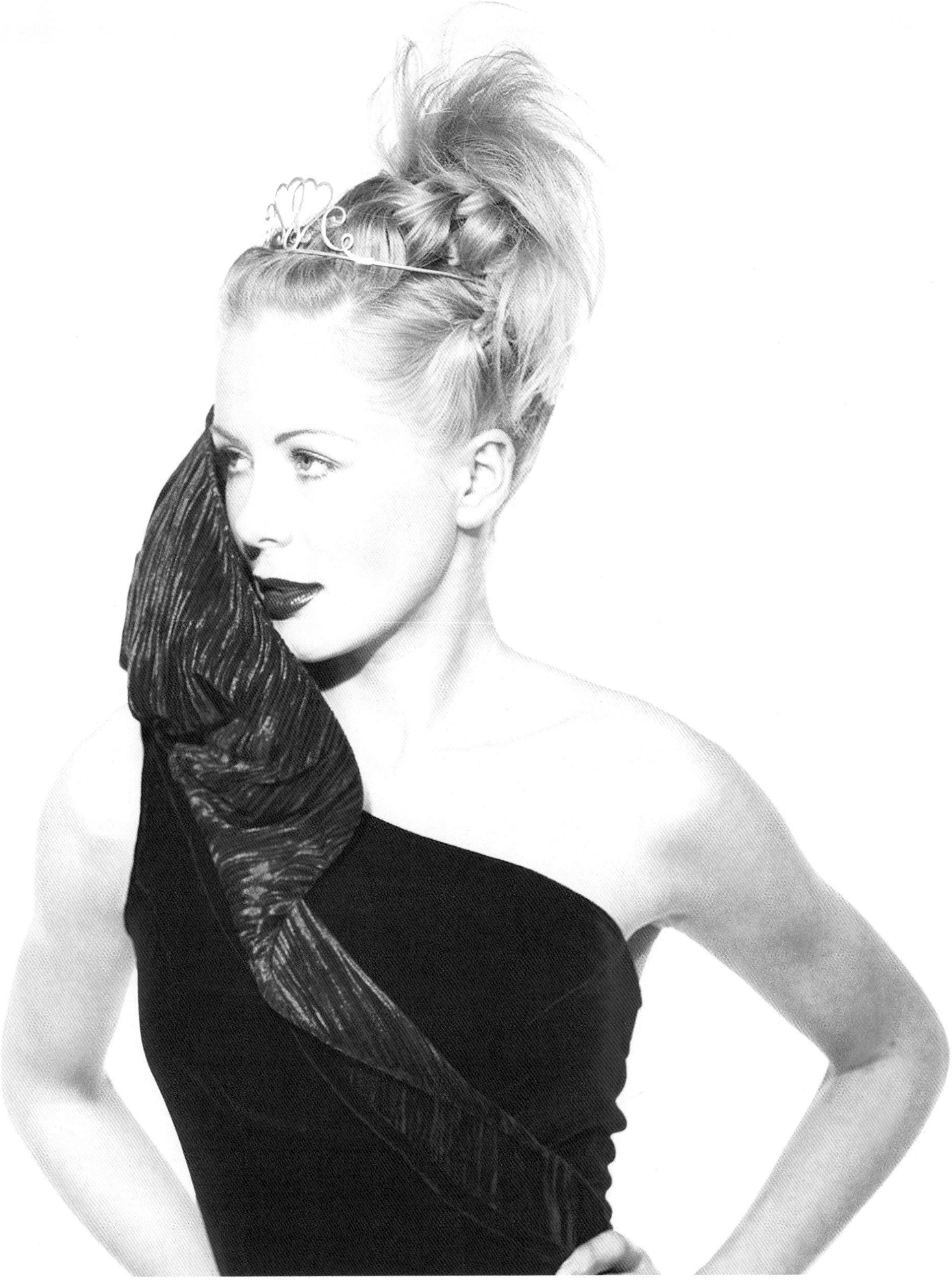

BACK TO THE FUTURE

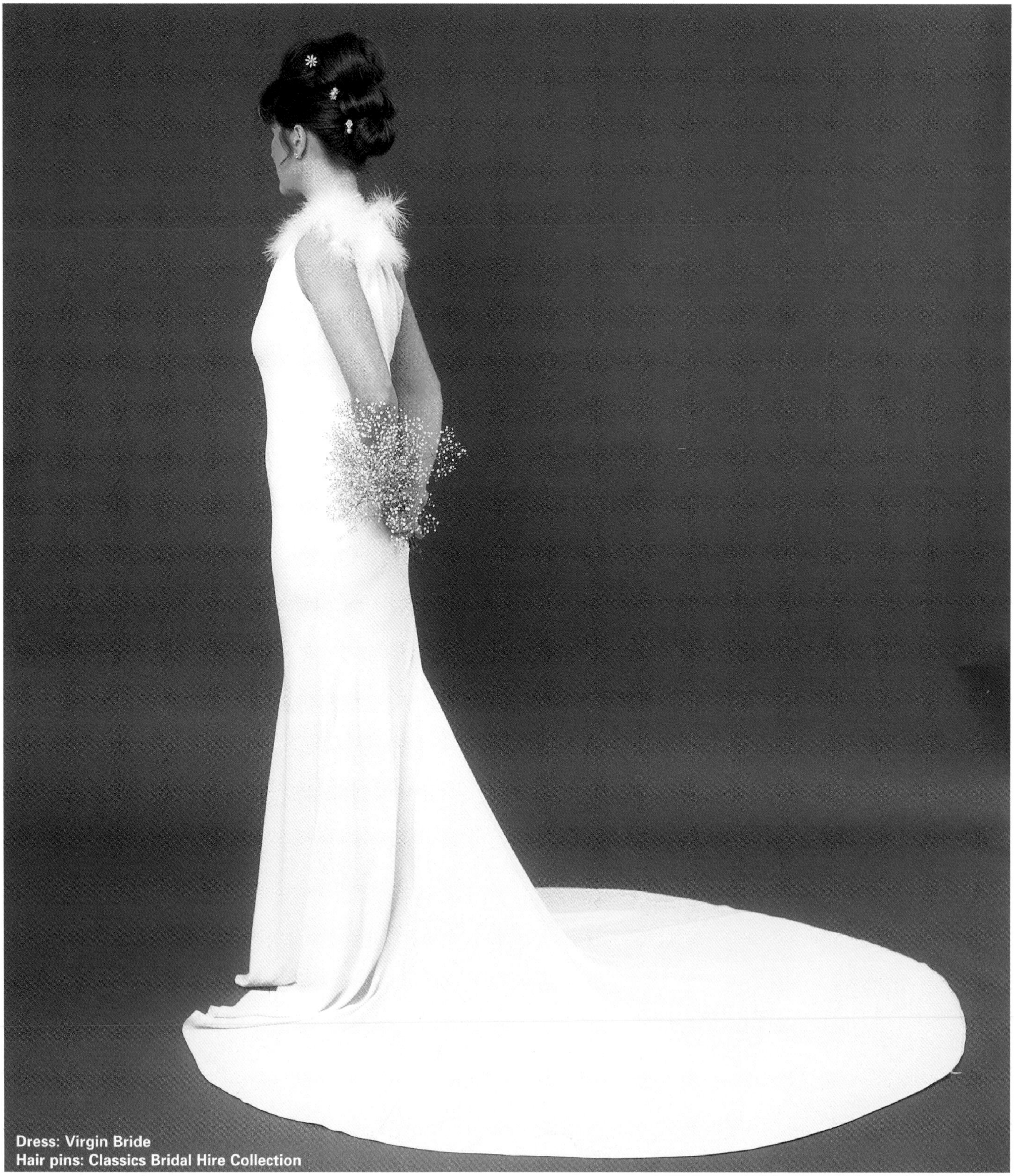

Dress: Virgin Bride
Hair pins: Classics Bridal Hire Collection

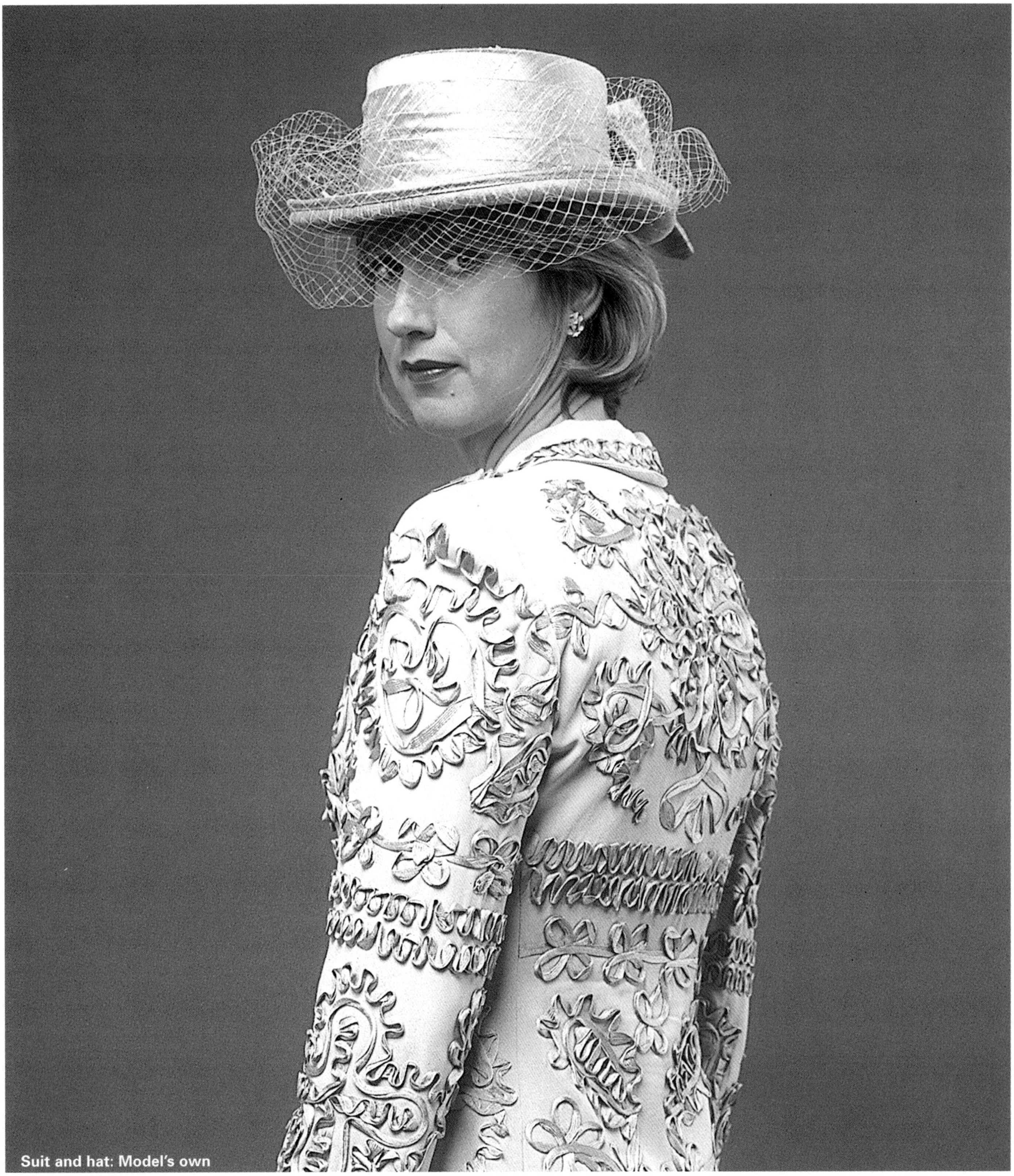

Suit and hat: Model's own

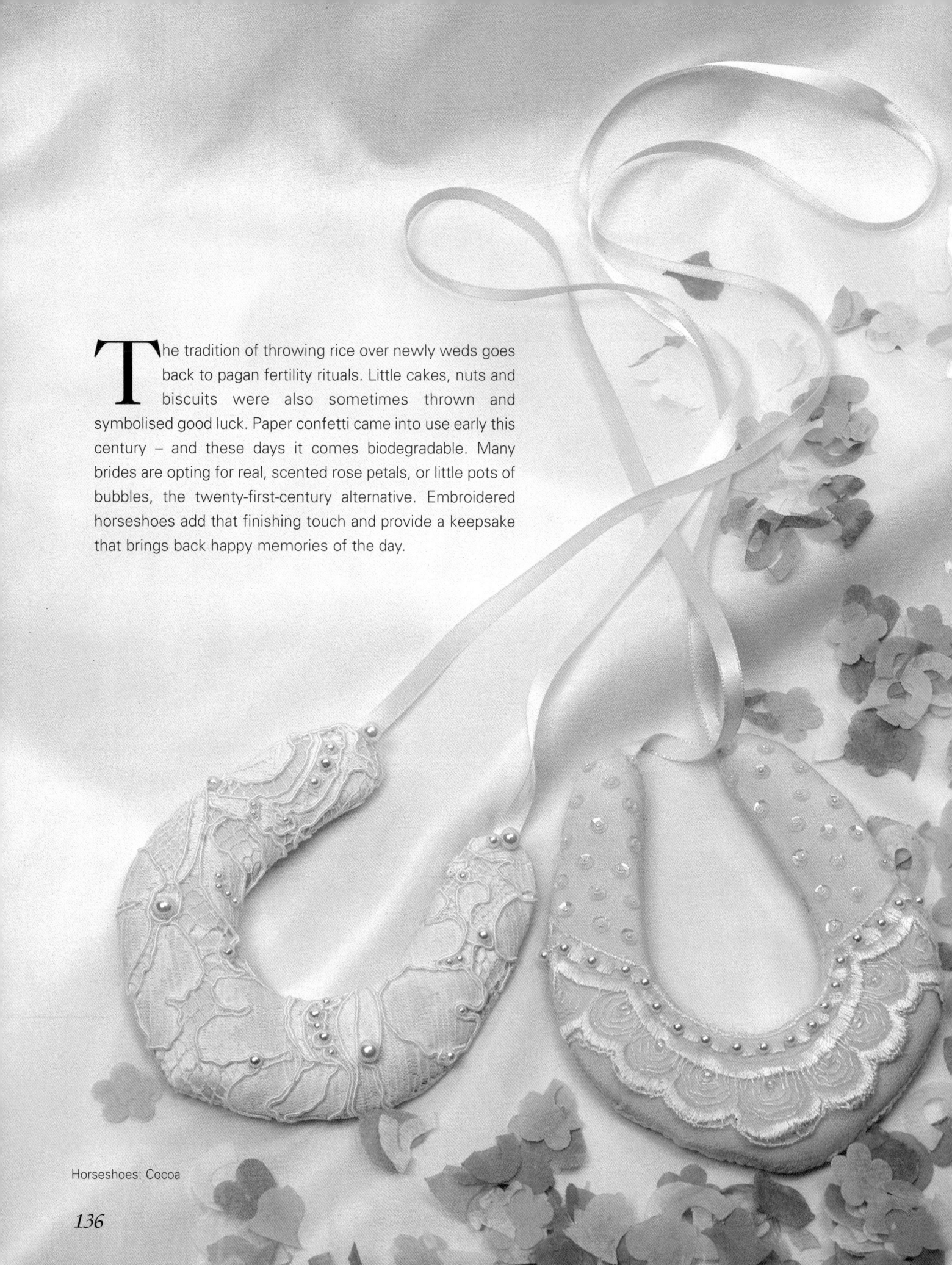

The tradition of throwing rice over newly weds goes back to pagan fertility rituals. Little cakes, nuts and biscuits were also sometimes thrown and symbolised good luck. Paper confetti came into use early this century – and these days it comes biodegradable. Many brides are opting for real, scented rose petals, or little pots of bubbles, the twenty-first-century alternative. Embroidered horseshoes add that finishing touch and provide a keepsake that brings back happy memories of the day.

Horseshoes: Cocoa

136